Natural
Fertility

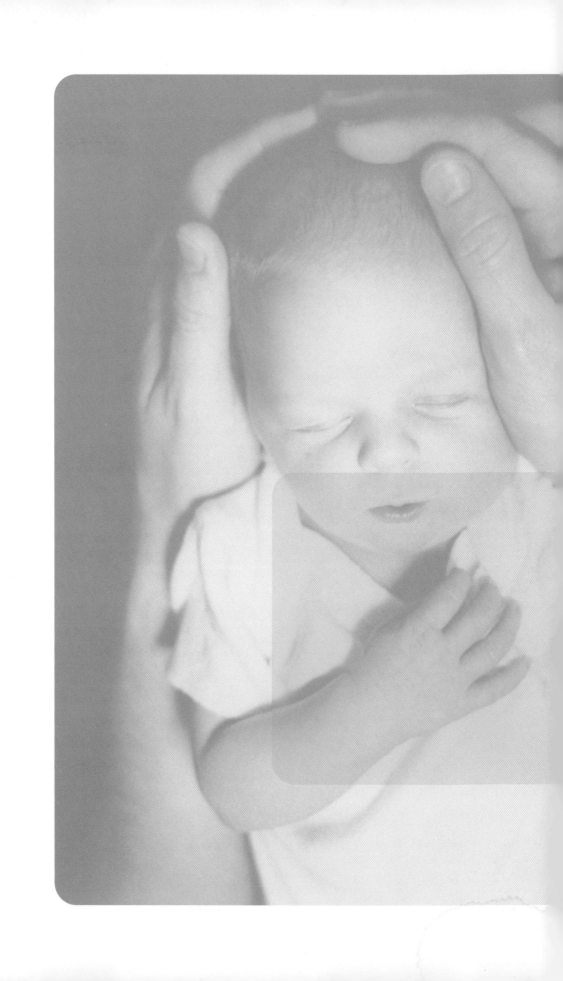

Natural Fertility

Nikki Bradford

hamlyn

THE AUTHOR

Nikki Bradford is an award-winning medical author and respected freelance health journalist. She has been Health Editor on several major national women's magazines, including *Good Housekeeping* and *Essentials*, and has written 11 other best-selling titles which have been published in America, Australia and Europe, including *The Hamlyn Encyclopedia of Complementary Health*, *The Miraculous World of your Unborn Baby*, *The Well Woman's Self Help Directory* and *Men's Health Matters*. Nikki is a member of The Royal Society of Medicine, was founding honorary secretary of The Guild of Health Writers and has two young children called Ben and Jessie.

First published in Great Britain in 2002 by Hamlyn, a division of Octopus Publishing Group Ltd
2-4 Heron Quays, London E14 4JP

Distributed in the United States and Canada by Sterling Publishing Co., Inc.
387 Park Avenue South, New York, NY 10016

Note
While the advice and information in this book are believed to be accurate and true at the time of going to press neither the author nor the publisher can accept any legal responsibility or liability for any errors or omissions that may be made. The reader should always consult a physician in all matters relating to health and particularly in respect of any symptoms which may require diagnosis or medical attention.

ISBN 0 600 60396 2

A CIP catalogue record for this book is available from the British Library

Printed and bound in China

10 9 8 7 6 5 4 3 2 1

Contents

Introduction 6

Fertility Facts: The Biology and Mechanics 8
- The truth about the best time to have sex • How much ages really matter
- Says who? Separating fertility facts from fiction • Reading your six secret
fertility signs • The Best – and worst – sex positions for getting pregnant
- Choosing your baby's gender • The science of ovulation and implantation

Self-help and Preconceptual Care 32
EVERYTHING YOU CAN DO TO MAXIMIZE YOUR OWN FERTILITY:
- Practical preconceptual care for women • Why your weight and exercise can
help • Bug-busting • Checking your emotional health • Which contraception
were you using? • Preconceptual care for men • Fertility foods • Detoxing
- The dangers of 'silver' tooth fillings • Stress and infertility – the full story
- Job hazards for future mothers and fathers • DIY, decorating, furnishings and
gardening • Medicines and street drugs

Complementary Therapies 76
HOW AND WHY THESE THERAPIES CAN HELP COUPLES BECOME PREGNANT:
- Homeopathy • Western herbalism • Ayurvedic medicine • Bach flower
remedies • Acupuncture • Acupressure • Chinese herbal medicine
- Aromatherapy • Reflexology • Hypnotherapy and self-hypnosis • Autogenic
training • Relaxation and visualization • Feng Shui

The Medical Side of Fertility Treatment 112
CAUSES AND TREATMENTS FOR FERTILITY PROBLEMS:
For Women • Ovulation disorders • Blocked Fallopian tubes • Polycystic
ovarian syndrome • Endometriosis • Sperm antibodies • Fibroids • Cervical
mucus disorders • Recurrent miscarriage • Blood clotting disorders • Genetics
For men • Semen problems • Retrograde ejaculation • Hormonal disorders
- Genetics and environmental factors
Plus • Negotiating the private fertility jungle

Pregnant? Hooray! 130

References 136

Editorial Consultants 138

Helplines 139

Index 140

Acknowledgements 144

Introduction

This book is for everyone, woman or man, who wants to have a baby. For anyone who:

- is just quietly thinking about it
- has just begun trying
- has been trying for months, or even years, with either no results or a history of miscarriages.

Losing confidence

Recent weighty clinical research insists that couples in the West are actually getting pregnant faster than ever before (without medical assistance too) because they know when their fertile time of the month is. Yet top European infertility experts have also recently gone on record saying that couples are losing faith in their own power to create pregnancy naturally and are making for expensive, private infertility clinics too soon.

Infertility is big business

An astonishing 1 in 80 British babies is now born with some help from a fertility lab, more in the USA, and in Scandinavia it's 1 in 50. Fertility is

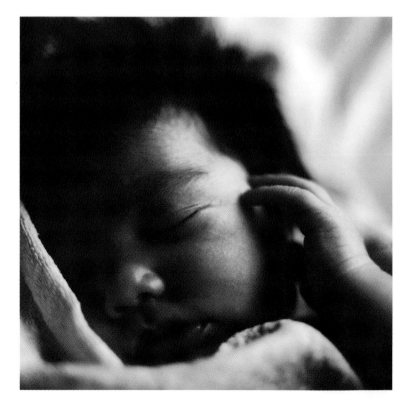

big business – IVF's price tag is now an average of £2,500 ($4,500) per try with 3–4 attempts considered usual. If there is a growth industry in medicine, this is it. Someone out there is making a lot of money out of our (apparently unjustified) lack of confidence.

Improving your chances of conceiving

Yet there is something more. Something very important that you may not have heard about. Two things, in fact. They are important because they well make all the difference between you being able to conceive easily and then carrying a healthy baby to term – and not.

YOU CAN MAXIMIZE YOUR OWN FERTILITY

The approach is called preconceptual care. Most of it is common sense and straightforward DIY lifestyle measures to get both the prospective mother and father into as healthy a state as possible before they begin to try for a baby. It involves detoxifying your system, taking mineral and vitamin supplements and adjusting your lifestyle so it is as stress free and healthy as possible. *You can see measurable results within just three to four months.*

COMPLEMENTARY THERAPY TREATMENTS FOR FERTILITY CAN REALLY WORK

They can work well if you have a good therapist who knows what he or she is doing. Reflexology, acupuncture, herbal medicine, nutrition and hypnosis – published medical research papers (see References, page 136) show these therapies can support and improve fertility in many ways, from helping a woman who is not releasing eggs to ovulate, to improving a man's sperm count and quality. Just as importantly, they can also help you cope with the considerable stress of trying for pregnancy – especially if it's taking longer than you had thought, or if you are having invasive, expensive medical fertility treatments.

It's you who chooses the therapy, you who chooses the therapist and you who works in partnership with that therapist instead of being a 'patient' to whom things are done. Complementary and orthodox medical treatments can also work very well indeed together. It does not have to be a case or either one or the other.

Putting you back in control

Preconceptual care and complementary therapies put you back in the driving seat and make the very most of your chances to conceive without extra help. They also maximize the likelihood of medical treatment working out for you should you need it after all.

This straightforward, sensible and natural dual approach has helped many thousands of couples become pregnant, cut their risk of miscarriage and have healthy babies.

It could help you too.

COMPLEMENTARY THERAPIES

Unlike medical fertility drugs and treatments, complementary therapies are gentle, very low on side-effects, and, for most people, affordable.

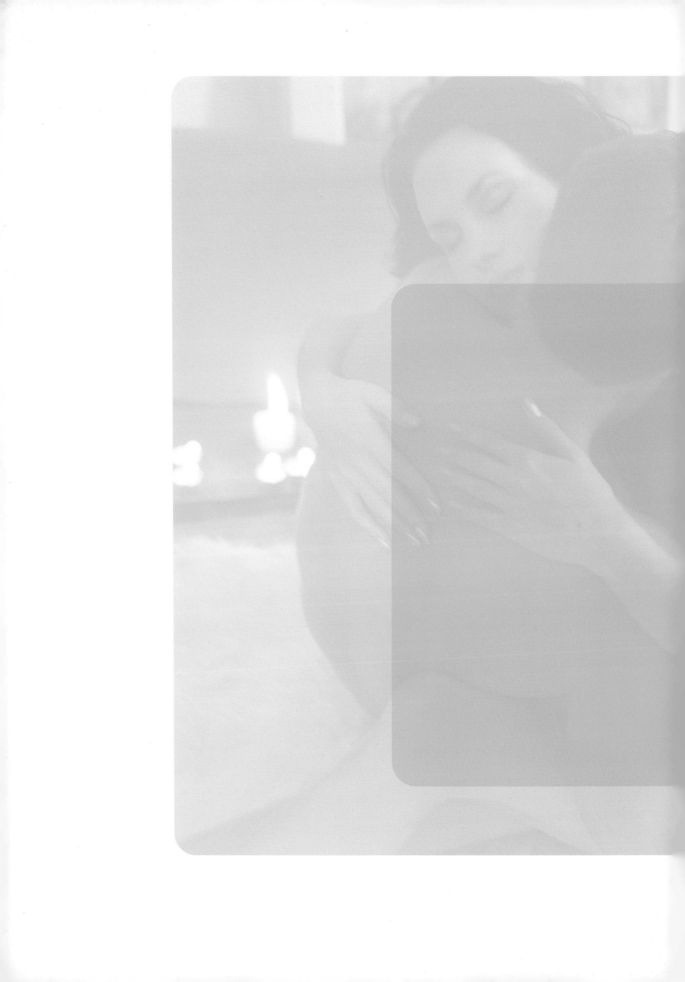

Fertility Facts:
The Biology and Mechanics

From the second you were both conceived, you and your partner have each been unique.

All human life begins from a single Mother Cell formed by the father's sperm and mother's ovum, and such are the possibilities of genetic variation that this cell contains a blueprint for life itself that is like no one else's, whoever has been born in the past or whoever will be born in the future.

That's how you started off, and that's how your own child will begin life, as a pinhead-sized bundle of possibilities. Understanding a bit about how your own reproductive system operates will help explain why your health can be so vital for being able to get pregnant in the first place, and having a healthy baby at the end of it.

Since even before you were born, your body has been equipping you for creating a conception of your own, forming and refining the biological systems that will make you fertile. If you now want to boost that fertility – and give the baby you both want to have the very best possible start in life – read on ...

When Should We Have Sex?

Advice about the best time to have sex if you want to become pregnant has always been highly prescriptive. Many couples grappling gamely with temperature charts, ovulation thermometers and suggestions to 'save up the sperm for a week' find that, instead of being a pleasure, sex becomes at best a chore – or, at worst, a source of considerable stress and argument. If there is one thing that kills libido, it is a sense of obligation.

Let's take a look at the basics first, before looking at alternative approaches to this question. In order to become pregnant, four things need to happen:

1 Good-quality sperm must reach the woman's womb and Fallopian tubes.
2 A healthy ripe egg must be produced and released by the woman's ovary.
3 One of the sperm needs to meet up with an egg and fertilize it.
4 The now-fertilized egg has to implant itself securely in the womb lining, and start growing.

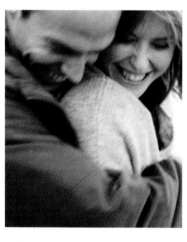

ABOVE Wanting to have a baby can intensify the romance in a relationship – even more for men than it does for women. A Gallup Poll in 1994 found that 23% of the women that were spoken to by researchers felt trying for a baby made sex even more special. The figure rose to 29% for would-be fathers, a further 1 in 20 of whom tentatively expressed the hope that it would encourage their partners to take the lead in bed.

Doctors have always told us that the best time for a woman to make love if she wants to get pregnant is the day her ripe egg is released from her ovary. Technically, that suggests a couple has to make love on one particular day a month (ovulation or 'O'-day) if they want to maximize their chances of having a baby.

We are also traditionally told that this day of days is right in the middle of a woman's menstrual cycle – around day 14 or 15, if her cycle lasts the 'classic' 28 days. The menstrual cycle is counted from the day one period begins all the way through to the first day of the next period. However, since only 20% or so of women have such a 28-day cycle, family-planning tutors have long advised couples to do the following simple sums to find out when the woman is ovulating:

'As a general guide, a woman will be fertile about 14 days before the date she expects her period to start. To calculate this time, take 14 days from the number of days between the start of one period and the start of the next. The resulting number will be the number of the day after the start of the period when the egg will be released, i.e. if there are 33 days between each period, the egg is released on 33–14=19 days from the start of the period.'
Infertility & Sex leaflet, CHILD, 1998

Adult numeracy must be a little better than the pessimistic national newspapers say, because couples who want to get pregnant have been conceiving more quickly than ever over the last ten years. Medical experts attribute this to us having a better understanding of when a woman's fertile period is. So – exactly two weeks before the day your next period is due is the time to have sex if you want to become pregnant. Right? Wrong! – according to two recent pieces of medical research which have revolutionized current thinking on fertility.

The truth about timing

The first, which was published in 2000 in the pages of the heavyweight *New England Journal of Medicine*, suggests that women are at their most fertile on both the day of ovulation and the day after that, as eggs live for up to 24 hours.

The second bombshell came from a study conducted by the US National Institute of Environmental Health Sciences (NIEH) in North Carolina, which suggested that fertility-day timing is far less predictable than experts had thought. Gynaecologists have always known that ovulation day can vary a little even for women with super-regular cycles, but they never realized how often this happened and to what extent. Now the NIEH study's figures suggest that, even in healthy women who have no fertility difficulties, *only one in three* ovulates between days 10 and 17 of their menstrual cycles, let alone on day 14.

This has caused a major stir in medical circles. But where does it leave couples who are not that bothered about the academic arguments, but just want to have a baby? (see Ovulation alert – the signs, page 24 and below).

Reading your body language

If you want to pinpoint your two or three days a month of peak fertility so you can time your lovemaking accordingly (without having to restrict it to one single day) it is worth being aware that a woman's body sends out several signals that you can easily learn to look for and recognize. The two most useful ones are:

- Changes in cervical mucus. There is more of it, and it is clear/ stretchy/slippery like egg white (see pages 23-24).
- Changes in body temperature. It falls sharply just before ovulation, then rises again and remains stable for the rest of the cycle.

No need to save up your sperm

Standard advice to would-be fathers wanting to maximize their chances of getting their partner pregnant has long been to save up sperm (that is don't ejaculate) for a week. Forget it. This approach doesn't work and never did because, while it may 'stack up' larger volumes of semen, it often reduces the quality of the sperm. If sperm are poorer in quality, they are less likely to make you pregnant no matter how many of them there are.

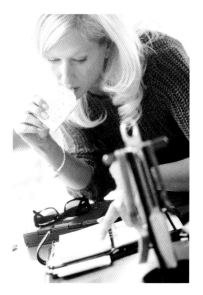

ABOVE Fertility experts have found women usually ovulate at 4pm. An excellent time to make love if you want to conceive therefore would be lunchtime (if you could find somewhere private to meet) which would certainly cheer up the average working day.

Does Age Really Matter?

The short answer, if you are both fit and healthy, is – it matters less than everyone thinks. Though the optimum time for a woman to conceive and go through pregnancy is any time from early to mid-twenties up to the age of 35, this is not a magical cut-off date, and for a healthy woman who is trying to become pregnant in her mid- to late thirties the outlook is good.

The number of 'older mothers' who have their babies when they are 35 or above, is rising fast. In 1989, one in ten British women was having a baby at 35+; in 1999 it had risen to one in seven. By 2002, it is estimated that as many as one in six babies will be born to older mothers.

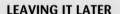

LEAVING IT LATER
Research suggests that in the UK 29% of women and 51% of men aged 18–34 are saying they want to delay having children for 'as long as possible'.

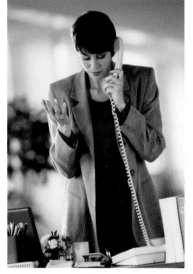

ABOVE One in 10 women say they have either had to considerably delay having children or had to give up their option to become a mother at all for the sake of their career.
(Survey 1998: *WFD Consultancy*, with *Management Today*)

RIGHT Between eight and nine couples out of ten in their twenties will conceive within a year of trying; between four and five couples out of ten who are over 40 will do so within a year. One major reason for the difference is the number of cycles women have per year when they actually ovulate fertile eggs – it doesn't happen every time. See chart, right.

For women

FERTILITY – HOW QUICKLY WILL I GET PREGNANT?

A woman's fertility does decline as she becomes older, but it's a slow process, which only accelerates as she reaches her later thirties. While it is true that a woman of, say, 25 has twice the likelihood of becoming pregnant each month as a woman of 37 or 38, and therefore is likely to conceive more quickly, the chances of the older woman doing so within

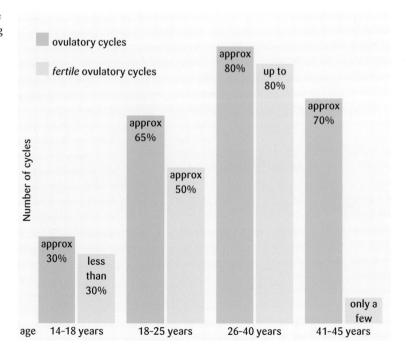

ovulatory cycles

fertile ovulatory cycles

Number of cycles

| age | 14–18 years | 18–25 years | 26–40 years | 41–45 years |

- 14–18 years: approx 30% / less than 30%
- 18–25 years: approx 65% / approx 50%
- 26–40 years: approx 80% / up to 80%
- 41–45 years: approx 70% / only a few

the year are also good. Looked at another way, eight or nine out of ten couples in their twenties will become pregnant within a year of beginning to try for a baby. For couples in their mid-thirties, it's about a seven in ten chance that they will conceive within the year. For women over the age of 40, four to five out of every ten will succeed in becoming pregnant within a year.

For women over the age of 45, only one in ten will become pregnant within a year. This is because in the ten years leading up to the menopause – the average age for which is 51 – most women only ovulate a ripe egg an average of eight times a year out of 11–14 menstrual cycles. And not all of these eggs are fertile anyway, or able to survive long enough for the pregnancy to become established and implant itself in the womb. Even if it does, the womb lining may be less receptive than a younger woman's because the levels of the hormones oestrogen and progesterone are likely to be lower.

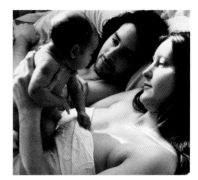

ABOVE Most babies are born normal and healthy, regardless of how old their parents are.

MISCARRIAGE AND OLDER MUMS

The majority (60–70%) of confirmed pregnancies for mothers between 40 and 45 work out fine. Over the age of 45, the chances of a pregnancy going to term and resulting in a live baby are nearer 50%, and they become less as a woman becomes older.

Older mothers certainly do run more of a risk of miscarrying than younger ones. According to Dr Richard Aubry, professor of obstetrics and gynaecology at the State University of New York, the chances of miscarriage are around 10–12% for the under 35s; then about 15% for 35–40 year olds, roughly 20% for 40 year olds and nearer 25% for women aged 43–45. Over the age of 45, it can be as high as 45%.

WILL MY BABY BE NORMAL?

In the majority of cases for women of all ages, the answer to this question is a resounding 'Yes'. Taking account of all the babies born to mothers of all ages right across the board in the UK, 98% are completely normal and healthy. And, of those who are born with what doctors call a birth 'defect', in many cases it is something minor and correctable like a smallish birthmark or a slight squint.

However, ovaries do get older along with the rest of the body, and as they do so the risk of genetic problems increases. Studies suggest that for women over the age of 35 one in every three eggs is in some way less than perfect. This means that 'older' women are more likely than younger ones to have a pregnancy affected by chromosomal problems, and are therefore more likely to miscarry.

One example of this is Down's syndrome. The risk of conceiving a Down's baby is just 1 in 2,000 for a woman of 20. At 30, it is 1 in 800, at 35 it is 1 in 300, at 38 it is 1 in 180, at 40 it is 1 in 100 and at 45 it is 1 in 30. This is why an amniocentesis test, in which a small sample from the fluid surrounding the baby is taken out through a fine needle, is usually offered to all pregnant women over the age of 35. An amniocentesis test can detect 99% of all cases of Down's syndrome.

HOW LONG HAVE I GOT?
The easiest time to get pregnant lasts for longer than most of us realize – it's between the ages of 25 and 38.

DOWN'S SYNDROME

Although an older mother has a greater risk of conceiving a baby who has Down's syndrome, a younger mother is, in fact, more likely to give birth to one. This is because women who are statistically more at risk, that is those over 35, usually choose to have an amniocentesis test and will often elect to terminate the pregnancy if they find out that the child they are carrying is affected. However, younger women tend not to go for the amniocentesis option because their risk is far smaller, so the presence of the syndrome remains undetected until after the birth.

In recent years a new check has been developed that can be done at the same time as a routine ultrasound at around 16–18 weeks. This looks at an area at the back of the baby's neck called the nuchal fold. In babies with Down's syndrome this is temporarily thickened, which can give an indication of whether a baby is affected without needing to use amniocentesis. If the nuchal fold check becomes standard procedure and is looked at as a matter of course along with the usual things like the baby's head circumference and limb measurements, it could help to identify affected babies for younger women too.

The likelihood of Down's syndrome can also be predicted by a screening check in the form of a basic blood test called the alpha-fetoprotein (AFP) test. The AFP test is carried out around 16 weeks into the pregnancy and, although it doesn't give a definite answer, it does give a likelihood rating of possible problems such as Down's and spina bifida (an abnormality in development of the head or spine). If it is 'positive', this doesn't mean there definitely is something wrong, merely that there may be, and that the mother would benefit from a more accurate diagnostic test such as amniocentesis to check up for sure.

For men

Most men over the age of 50 begin to undergo testicular failure, that is their sperm count starts to drop.

THE ANDROPAUSE

The andropause, also known as the viropause, is thought to be a physical phenomenon similar to the menopause in that it has many similar symptoms and is caused by a drop in available-for-use sex hormones. In the men's case this is testosterone, rather than oestrogen or progesterone. The andropause is not the same as the male 'mid-life crisis' (the male menopause), which most psychologists and psychiatrists agree exists to some degree, but which is thought to be more of an emotional phenomenon.

Dr Malcolm Carruthers, formerly head of pathology services at London's Maudesley Hospital and now medical director of the Positive Health Centre in Harley Street, London, has researched this area for the last 15 years. In that time he has gathered sufficient scientific evidence to back up his belief that the andropause is a physical phenomenon, which hits 'perhaps 25% of 50 year olds and 40% of 60 year olds'.

Based on initial research with one thousand apparently andropausal patients, Dr Carruthers found striking parallels with a woman's menopause. These included night sweats, irritability, drier skin, low-level depression, changes in gender-pattern body hair on the chest and arms, and less of a 5 o'clock shadow if the man used to notice one. The men also reported reduced sexual desire and loss of drive in general.

These symptoms may be due to lower levels of free testosterone circulating in the blood. This is not the same as lower general levels of testosterone per se. The reasons for having less circulating testosterone are not straightforward, and may include a problem with the cells that make testosterone (the Leydig cells) or with the pituitary gland. According to Dr Sammy Lee of the Portland Hospital's Fertility Unit in London who has been studying hormone levels in men with reproductive problems for 15 years, when the testes fail they get smaller and atrophy but still produce high levels of usable testosterone. They may be 'peri-andropausal' (like peri-menopausal – the time leading up to the menopause) for up to seven years before failing totally, and then testosterone levels certainly will plummet.

Blood tests offered by doctors who believe in the existence of the andropause can check for a man's levels of the hormone called follicle-stimulating hormone (FSH). They look at this rather than at testosterone itself because FSH stimulates the testes to make sperm. They also check levels of luteinizing hormone, or LH, which encourages testosterone production. Any problems with the levels of these vital male sex hormones can affect fertility and libido. 'Anything that affects a man's ability to produce active testosterone is going to affect his fertility too,' says Dr Carruthers.

Treatments include stopping smoking, taking more exercise, drinking less alcohol, stress-busting/relaxing measures and, if all else fails, male hormone replacement therapy (HRT), which involves regular doses of testosterone. The latter is usually expensive and should not be offered as a first line of treatment. If he is taking male HRT, a man also needs to have a detailed ultrasound scan and blood test to check for underlying prostate cancer every six months. This is because testosterone may encourage any predisposition to prostate cancer in older men (that is over the age of 50).

MEN HAVE A BIOLOGICAL CLOCK TICKING TOO

It has always been thought that the biological clock theory only applied to women, but recent research by Bristol and Brunel Universities in the UK involving 8,500 couples has revealed that the older a man is the longer it will usually take for him to get his partner pregnant, regardless of how old she is.

One possible reason for this is the likelihood of an increased number of genetic errors in the sperm as the man ages. The older man is more likely to have suffered from an infection affecting sperm production or tube patency, or to have been adversely affected by either environmental toxins or work conditions.

> **THE DIFFERENCE BETWEEN DECADES**
> A 35-year-old man's likelihood of taking over a year to get his partner pregnant is twice what it would be if he were 25 years old. The chances of a couple conceiving within six months of trying for a baby drop by 2% each year after a man passes the age of 24.

A FATHER'S AGE AND POSSIBLE BIRTH DEFECTS

In general, there is little connection between birth defects or disorders and a baby's father's age. However, there are a few exceptions.

According to a study in British Columbia of 10,000 babies born between 1952 and 1973, older fathers appeared to have slightly more children affected by specific conditions such as congenital cataracts and Down's syndrome. Men over 50 were also found to be twice as likely as men aged 25–29 to have a baby with spina bifida. However, as 1 in 600 conceptions is affected by this condition anyway, that gives a risk of 1 in 300.

> **CUT CHOLESTEROL**
> If a man's arteries have become furred up with plaque (a mixture of calcium and cholesterol) or have hardened – as commonly occurs in older men – they become narrower and less blood can get through. Poor blood supply can reduce the production of testosterone in the testes.

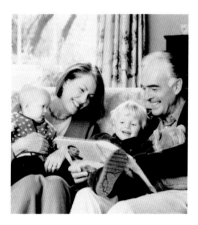

ABOVE Women with older partners often say older men are better fathers than younger men because they are calmer, have more experience of life, are more secure in their own identity and may have had children before.

> **80-YEAR-OLD FATHERS**
> The normal range of testosterone levels in men is very wide and some 70 year olds can have levels equal to some 24-year-old men. However, generally, an 80 year old can still father children even though he has only half the testosterone of a 30 year old, suggesting that testosterone levels alone are not that important.

PHOTOCOPYING ERRORS IN SPERM

Sperm are more likely to be faulty than eggs. This is because they go through an estimated 380 cell divisions before they become an adult tadpole-shaped cell ready for action, and each time a cell divides genetic copying errors can occur. There is far less opportunity for error with a woman's egg cell, since only about 23 cell divisions are needed to create one.

The probability of certain other rare genetic disorders, such as Marfan's syndrome (an inherited disorder characterized by abnormal tallness) and malformations of the skull, hands and feet, rises slightly with a father's age, and the risk of achondroplasia (dwarfism) also increases, though it remains rare. There also appears to be a link between schizophrenia and a father's age. A report published in 2001 by the New York University School of Medicine and the Israeli Ministry of Health suggests that new fathers between 45 and 50 are twice as likely as new fathers under 25 to have children with schizophrenia.

OLDER FATHERS AND MISCARRIAGE RISK

Women with much older partners are more likely to have miscarriages. This is because babies who are conceived when a damaged sperm fertilizes the egg are often miscarried in the earliest part of pregnancy, and older men tend to have more abnormal sperm. These may have an overly large or too-small head, two heads, or a tendency to swim around in circles.

Fortunately, most men can make significant improvements in their sperm quality by taking some straightforward DIY measures, such as stopping smoking (see pages 47–48), changing their diet (see pages 53–54), taking exercise, and even – yes, the rumours about tight underpants are true – looking to their choice of underwear (see page 48).

GENETIC COUNSELLING – DO YOU WANT TO TALK TO SOMEONE?

You may like to consider genetic counselling if you are at all concerned about the possible effects of your age on your fertility (doctors reckon a woman who is 40+ or a man who is 50+ is a medically 'older' parent) or the health of your future baby. Other reasons for consulting a genetic counsellor are if you have had several miscarriages or a previous stillbirth or if you have an older child with an inherited disorder and you think there may be an inherited illness in your family.

A genetic counsellor is usually a doctor with specialist training in inherited diseases that can be passed from one generation to the next via a tiny fault in a gene. He or she will want to find out as much as possible about all children born on both sides of your families going back over the previous three generations. If there is a strong likelihood of a gene disorder affecting your pregnancy, you may be offered genetic testing (screening). Such inherited gene disorders include dwarfism, cystic fibrosis, haemophilia, Fragile X syndrome and Duchenne muscular dystrophy.

Ovulation, Conception and Fertilization

Inside a woman's body

During her fertile years, a woman's body gets ready for a possible pregnancy once a month. Two main things happen: the lining of her womb (endometrium) thickens until it is as lush and welcoming as it can possibly be should a fertilized egg happen to come along, and one of her ovaries will ripen and release an egg (occasionally two eggs). This happens less often when a woman first starts to have periods, and becomes less frequent again when she reaches her mid-thirties and (especially) early forties.

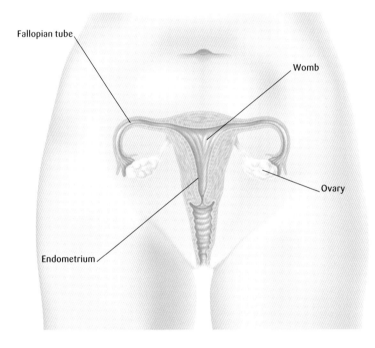

Fallopian tube

Womb

Ovary

Endometrium

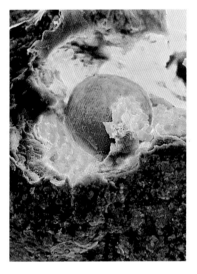

ABOVE A ripened egg breaking free from its nest in the ovary follicle. The biggest cell in the human body, it is the size of a grain of dust and is just visible to the naked eye.

LEFT Extraordinary as it may sound, as a woman you existed inside your own mother's – and your grandmother's – womb in the form of an unripened egg. Now your own daughters, and their daughters, exist in your womb in the same form.

Inside a man's body

From mid- to late puberty onwards, a man will be constantly making, maturing and storing millions of sperm in a process that takes between 80 and 100 days to complete. These sperm are produced in the testes in response to the male sex hormone testosterone and a number of other hormones.

Sperm are the cellular equivalent of Formula One racing cars. Lean and honed, they are nothing

VIVE LA DIFFERENCE
Men produce around 1,000 sperm cells every second (nearly 100 million a day). Women have around 10,000 unripe eggs at puberty and ripen roughly one a month in their fertile years.

TURBO-POWERED

Some 'turbo-charged' sperm can reach the Fallopian tubes, down which the eggs travel on their way from the ovary to the womb, in five minutes flat. Yet others are still arriving 'late but live' in the tubes several days later. This means a man's sperm is capable of getting a woman pregnant up to five days after making love. The message here is that your lovemaking does not have to occur on a certain day to result in pregnancy – there's plenty of leeway.

more than a nucleus carrying genetic information (the driver), energy-producing bodies called mitochondria (the fuel tank) and a long whiplash tail (the engine), which is five times the length of the nucleus head. When a man climaxes during intercourse, an average of 250 million sperm – roughly four times the population of Britain – are fired into the woman's vagina.

Semen is a vibrant mixture of:

- sperm cells – about 20% by volume;
- fluid from the man's seminal vesicle glands containing the fuel (fructose, a form of sugar) that gives the sperm the energy to swim up through the womb into the Fallopian tubes and break into a waiting egg if they are the first there. This accounts for about 70% of semen volume;
- fluid from two sex glands, the prostate and the Cowper's glands. These are alkaline and so help to neutralize some of the acidity of the woman's vagina, and the prostate fluid contains vital enzymes, proteins and minerals.

One question which couples often ask is whether it matters if some of the semen trickles back out of the vagina after lovemaking – don't you need all of it? In fact, you don't. This may seem strange when such emphasis is put on the number of sperm cells in a man's semen (the sperm count). However, it is perfectly normal for anything up to 90% of the semen ejaculated into the vagina to drain back out again afterwards. This happens because it changes its consistency once it is inside the warmth of the vagina. Semen is ejaculated in a soft gel form – probably to protect the sperm during ejaculation – but after a period of five to fifteen minutes inside the woman's body it liquifies, allowing the sperm to become mobile.

RIGHT Around 100 of the fittest sperm will reach the waiting egg, where a free-for-all ensues to be the first to break inside it. Immediately afterwards rapid changes take place in the outer membrane of the egg barring entrance to all others.

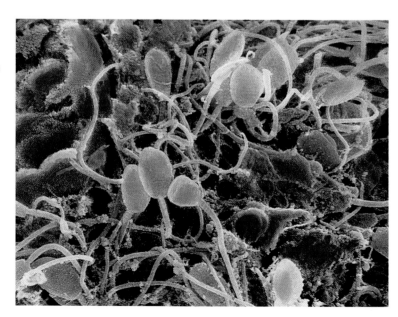

If you are concerned about the loss of semen after lovemaking, your doctor could arrange a simple check called a post-coital test (see page 117) to confirm whether the sperm cells are indeed managing to reach your womb and Fallopian tubes.

The three-step challenge

The sperm's first test is to stand up against the acidic environment of the vagina. Here they are given some protection by the fluid they swim in.

The second challenge is to power through the mucus that lies across the entrance to the cervical canal (the cervical os) that leads into the womb. Luckily, around a woman's ovulation time her body is programmed to give the sperm all the help it can. For example, in the days leading up to ovulation, a woman's cervical mucus becomes so sperm-friendly that it makes tiny 'go-faster' channels for the sperm to swim up.

> **SCENTSATIONAL**
> It is thought that a ripe egg releases an irresistible come-and-get-me scent to encourage sperm to hurtle towards it.

> **BLAST-OFF**
> Sperm are ejaculated from a man's body at about 16 kilometres per hour (10 mph). Fortunately, they are tough – they have to be. This speed may not sound like much to us. But to something as tiny as a sperm cell it may seem the equivalent of a novice passenger in a space rocket blasting away from earth's orbit at the speed of light, battered by unfeasibly high G forces.

By the time the sperm reach the egg, it is usually coming down the Fallopian tubes, stroked gently along by tiny fronds called cilia. If you look at a cross-section of Fallopian tube, these fronds make it look like a beautiful sea anemone.

Only about 100 of the fastest and fittest sperm troopers will survive the journey up through the womb and into the Fallopian tubes. The winner is the one that beats its rivals to the egg's surface and manages to break inside before they do.

Getting into the egg is the sperm's third challenge. It is able to do so because each one has a tiny bag of enzymes on the front of its 'head'

LEFT Here is a sperm cell powering inside the egg's 'shell'. It does so by means of a tiny bag of potent enzymes called the acrosome, which it carries on its head like the bumper on a sports car. This bag bursts open as it crashes into the egg's surface and the chemicals it contains dissolve a small part of the egg's shell, creating a small gap for the sperm to wriggle through.

called an acrosome. When it crashes into the egg's surface, this bag bursts open like an exploding chemical warhead, dissolves part of the egg's protective shell and makes an opening big enough for the sperm to wriggle through by furiously lashing its tail from side to side. As soon as it is through, changes take place in the egg's surface, barring entrance to all other sperm.

Fertilization

Once safely inside, the genetic material of the sperm cell's nucleus (the contents of its 'head') merges with that of the egg to create a Mother Cell. Over the next 24 hours, 23 pairs of chromosomes are formed, as one set of 23 from the sperm and another set of 23 from the egg combine. Once this has happened, your bundle of two merged cells is biologically a future baby, and known as an embryo until it is eight weeks old. After eight weeks it is known as a fetus.

DID YOU KNOW?
It wasn't until 1678 (after the invention of the microscope) that scientists cottoned on to the idea that sperm contained the seeds of life, though they thought each one contained a very miniature baby. And it took another 150 years before a Dutch microscopist called Antoni van Leeuwenhoek 'discovered' the egg, or ovum.

THE MAKING OF TWINS
If a woman has ovulated two ripe eggs instead of one and they are both fertilized (by different sperm), non-identical, or fraternal, twins can result. They may be a boy and a girl, two boys or two girls, and other than their age, will be no more alike than any other two siblings.

Twins can also be created when a single egg-and-sperm fertilized bundle of genetic material splits in half at a very early stage. This creates identical twins, consisting of two babies of the same sex with the same genetic make-up.

Non-identical twins are more common than identical twins, and can run in families. About 1 in 80 babies these days is a twin, up from 1 in 100 15 years ago. It is thought that the rise in numbers may be partly because more women are having assisted fertility treatments. These involve medications that stimulate their ovaries to release more than one egg at a time. Also, more couples are having *in-vitro* fertilization (IVF) treatment, in which eggs are fertilized outside the body and the embryos then placed inside the mother's womb. With IVF, more than one embryo is placed in the womb at a time; in fact, the average is from two to four.

Implantation and the Very First Few Days

Once the egg is fertilized, two more important things need to happen before a woman becomes properly pregnant. The first is that the tiny embryo needs to spend the next few days growing while it floats down the Fallopian tube and into the womb. In fact, it will be developing from a single cell housing two nuclei into a 64-cell structure called a morula.

The second is that the morula must then burrow its way into the womb lining, and attach itself there unshakeably.

The process of turning a successful fertilization into a pregnancy usually takes anything from five to eight days. By day seven the morula, which has grown larger and developed a shell (and which embryologists now call a blastocyst) begins to sprout small fronds from its surface; these are called chorionic villi. These help it to embed into any surface it lands on.

The surface concerned is almost always the rich lining of the womb, which the female body faithfully prepares each month for just such an occasion. However, every so often (1 in 200 cases) the embryo attaches itself to the lining of the Fallopian tube instead. When it begins to develop there, this is known as an ectopic pregnancy and it cannot last long since there is so little room – the inside of a Fallopian tube is about as wide as a fine sewing needle.

An ectopic pregnancy is more likely if one tube is partially blocked, perhaps by a previous infection. If you suspect that an early pregnancy may not be developing in the right place (symptoms include sharp abdominal pain), go to the hospital emergency department without delay and ask for a scan. This will either reassure you that all is well, or enable doctors to arrange for immediate treatment. It is vital that an ectopic pregnancy is dealt with right away. Treatment usually entails surgical removal of the pregnancy and careful repair or removal of the tube concerned.

Assuming that it makes it past the Fallopian tube, by day eight or so the little embryo will have floated down into the womb. It then anchors itself to the womb lining (usually on the upper back wall) by releasing chemicals that eat away a tiny area of lining, creating a burrow for the embryo to make its home in. If it manages this, congratulations – you are now officially pregnant!

The embryo's vigorous burrowing provides it with its first meal: a nourishing mixture of sugars, fats, proteins and other vital nutrients. This provides the energy for the development of seeker fronds which can tap into the tiny blood vessels, or capillaries, supplying the womb's lining, just like a tiny new plant sends out roots to search for water.

TINY BUT TOUGH
By day 4 the embryo is 16 cells big and the size of a pin tip.

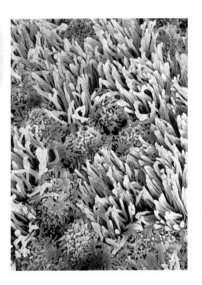

ABOVE This may look like a slice of exotic coral reef life, but it's a magnified picture of the inside of a Fallopian tube. The sea-anemone-like fronds are called cilia, which help stroke the egg down the length of the Fallopian tube and into the womb. The purple spongy areas are the tube's secretory cells which make a special fluid that protects, feeds and nurtures the egg on its journey.

WHEN WILL YOU KNOW YOU ARE PREGNANT?

You won't be able to get a true result from a pregnancy test until the first day after you expected your period to arrive. However, many women say they just knew from the moment their egg was fertilized. According to the traditional Chinese medical texts, there are signs immediately after sex that the woman has conceived – her desire is completely satiated, her body is exhausted and it feels very heavy.

Blood flows from these capillaries into the spaces at the thickening base of the embryo and back out again into the mother's veins. The base also starts to grow inwards, sending out more minute tendrils into the womb lining and, later on, into the body of the womb itself. This gradually forms the growing baby's placenta, the lifeline that brings food and oxygen from the mother's system, and takes away waste products.

The influential embryo

The embryo is enormously powerful for something so tiny – so powerful that it stops the woman having a period as normal and losing the pregnancy. Even before it manages to embed itself in the womb lining, it has been sending out chemical messengers to the mother's body in order to help itself survive.

One of the most important of these is the hormone called human chorionic gonadotrophin (HCG). HCG stimulates the egg capsule in the ovary, which originally ripened then released the egg, to keep making the sex hormone progesterone. The extra progesterone stops menstruation and the shedding of the womb lining, thus preserving the embryo's environment and keeping the very early pregnancy safe.

However, the process is not quite as easy as it sounds, and, although about a quarter of the embryos do manage to anchor themselves safely, it is thought that up to three-quarters of very early conceptions do not work out and are lost without the mother even knowing that she was pregnant at all.

RIGHT This is a four-day-old (16-cell) embryo – a potential human being who, at the moment, fits perfectly onto the tip of an ordinary pin.

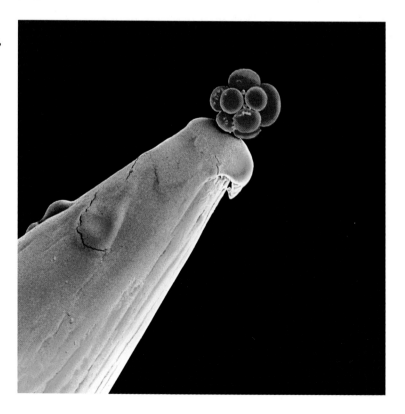

How to Read Your Own Fertility Signs

Would you say the workings of your body were a bit of a mystery to you, or are you pretty much aware of most of the changes it goes through?

Although many women are unaware of it, the female body constantly sends out a series of secret signals to tell her when she is at her most fertile. Some women find these easier to spot than others, but with practice and support every woman can learn to read her own body's sign language and understand a bit more about what is going on 'down there'. These signs can be invaluable markers to tell you the best days to try for a baby.

The amazing cervix

First, it may help to have some information about one of the main players – the cervix – and what it does. The cervix is a curved hemisphere of muscular tissue about 2 cm (1 in) in diameter when closed, which nestles right up at the top of the vagina farthest from the entrance. If you slide a clean finger inside the vagina and feel gently around at the top end, you will be able to detect this bump with the texture of satin, which guards the entrance to the womb. It changes quite dramatically depending on which hormones are being made and on the stage of the menstrual cycle.

The cervix is a remarkable feat of biological design because it has a wide range of different jobs:

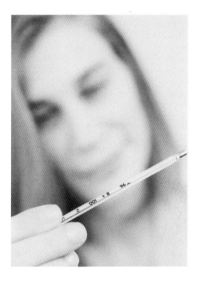

ABOVE Taking your temperature for fertility purposes is made considerably easier if you use a special thermometer with large numbers and gradients on it. They are available from natural family planning and fertility awareness organizations (see Helplines page 139).

- It separates and protects the womb from the outside world, preventing any germs from entering.
- It opens slightly each month to allow menstrual blood to flow out during your periods.
- It remains closed in pregnancy and withstands the weight of the growing baby until it is time for the child to be born.
- It stretches gently during childbirth, creating a channel big enough to allow a baby's head to pass through.
- It makes different types of mucus depending on the time of the month. This can be designed to lubricate the area, to help protect sperm when they arrive, or to keep them at bay. This last role is especially important in helping you become pregnant.

The cervix has a slim channel running through it called the cervical canal. This passageway, which is normally about 2–3 cm (1–1¼ inches) long and 1 mm (¹⁄₂₅ inch) across – but expands to over 10 cm (4 inches) across during childbirth – leads up into the inside of the womb itself. The canal is lined with special mucus-secreting glands. It is these which make the different types of secretions throughout the menstrual cycle. These are

SEXY SCENT
The cervix sends out three important signals during or just before ovulation (see page 24). However, the most noticeable one is usually an increase in clear vaginal mucus. Many men say this smells 'sexy and wonderful', probably because of the pheromones and high level of oestrogen it contains. The extra lubrication makes the woman feel damper or more slippery than usual around the entrance to the vagina.

WHEN TO MAKE LOVE
The latest - and most practical - advice on getting pregnant is to simply make love on any of the days that you notice more slippery mucus than usual. This is likely to be your most fertile time of the month.

clear and stretchy around ovulation time. At other times they are thicker and cream-coloured to protect any germs or environmental irritants from finding their way into the womb.

Ovulation alert - the signs

Certain key signals that occur during the menstrual cycle suggest that ovulation - and the days of peak fertility time - are very near. Many women find point No. 1 easiest to notice and it is probably the most important indicator of all. You may find you do not experience some of the others - such as No. 2 and No. 3 - at all.

1   **Fertile mucus**. This is clear, watery, stretchy mucus, like runny egg white. It is the most important fertility sign of all, and the easiest one to detect. Note: If you have a vaginal infection such as thrush, this can affect your mucus and you may not be able to see the fertility changes in it. It's important to get any infections like this treated before you try for a baby.

2   **Softer cervix**. It feels softer and less firm if you touch it gently with your finger. It will probably feel slippery with fertile mucus and its 'dimple' (os) opens a little until it is big enough to put the tip of your finger into gently. You may also notice, if you feel its position with your finger, that it has moved across slightly so it is right in the middle of the topmost part of the vagina, rather than slightly to one side of it.

3   **Ovulation pain**. Many women sometimes feel this as a dull ache on one side of the abdomen low down, and some even feel a sharpish pain. This can be a brief twinge or it can last the whole day and well into the evening.

4   **A tiny loss of blood**. This is not so common and, if you do notice it, it would be as well to check with your doctor that your cervix is healthy before definitely attributing it to ovulation.

5   **Feeling sexier**. Many women report a definite upsurge in their desire for sex around ovulation, and notice that it decreases again in the non-fertile days leading up to menstruation.

6   **Temperature**. Body temperature is affected by many things, including a change in levels of sex hormones. It cannot tell a woman when she is about to ovulate, but it will indicate that she has already done so. It drops slightly but steadily and noticeably until the time of ovulation, and soon afterwards it rises by around 0.2°C (0.4°F). If a woman charts her daily temperature for two to three months she will see the likely pattern of her fertility cycle, and it will help to predict when she is likely to ovulate. However, temperature

NO GUARANTEE
All the signs mentioned suggest that ovulation is likely, but none of them *guarantee* that it has occurred. In some cycles you will have signs of ovulation such as the clear mucus, but no egg is actually released. Some reports suggest that for women in their late thirties and early forties one-half to two-thirds of all cycles are anovulatory (that is they do not release a ripe egg).

charting can initially seem quite complicated, and it usually takes three to six months of practice to get used to it.

It may be useful to see a natural family planning counsellor who can help you to learn the temperature charting method. However, it is more usually used as a natural means of contraception rather than an aid to conception.

An ovulation prediction kit from the chemist can also be used to confirm your own natural indicators or if you are not quite sure that you are reading the signs correctly. The kits contain a simple dipstick urine test (usually five to a pack) which you can do at home. These work by detecting the upsurge of a hormone called luteinizing hormone (LH), which happens 24-36 hours before ovulation. However, ovulation prediction kits only pinpoint the LH surge - a positive result does not guarantee that an egg has actually been released. Note: If you have been diagnosed as having polycystic ovaries (see page 115) don't use these kits, because you will get inaccurate results.

THE SYMPTOTHERMAL CHART

You can use this temperature chart to help you work out when your more fertile times of the month are likely to be. It can be extended to make room for other indicators, such as the nature of your vaginal secretions, mucus quality, changes in your cervix and even mood changes.

| shortest cycle | 26 | start date | 26 March 2002 | route of temperature | oral X vaginal rectal | time of taking temperature | 7.30 am |

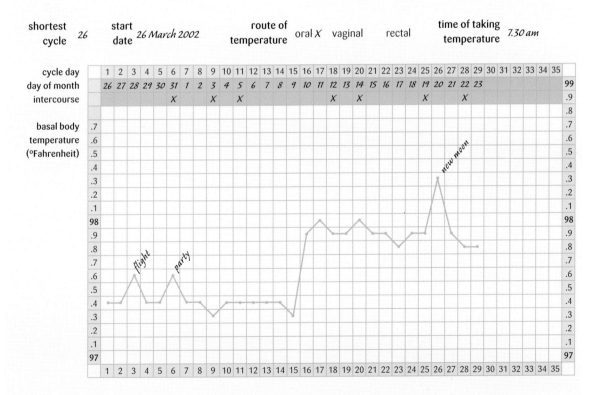

Says Who? Separating the Fertility Facts from the Fiction

There are probably more myths about fertility than about any other area of medicine, except maybe pregnancy itself. Add to that the rich store of traditional Old Wives' Tales, and stories from kind friends who are positive they heard it somewhere, and it makes for a subject saturated with inaccurate information. None of which is a lot of help to couples who are anxious to conceive a baby.

Here, courtesy of some top obstetricians, experienced midwives, parents themselves and some of the battier sites on the Internet, are some of the biggest getting pregnant and fertility myths, along with a few 'how to get a boy/girl baby' tips, the truth behind them, and what may have sparked them off.

'Some sex positions are better than others for getting pregnant'

THE MISSIONARY POSITION

Many experts believe that the man-on-top missionary position has the best chance of getting you pregnant, but there are no definitive studies to prove this. The rationale is that this position allows for deep penetration so the man's sperm can be ejaculated as close to the cervix as possible. This gives the sperm cells a flying start on their long journey, as the closer they are to their goal (the ripe egg waiting in the Fallopian tube several centimetres further up inside the woman's body) the more likely they are to reach it.

PILLOW TALK

Placing a pillow under the woman's hips before lovemaking is also thought to help the sperm along, as the angle of her vagina is steeper and so encourages deeper penetration. This may help conception for the same reason as the missionary position.

REAR ENTRY

If the man enters the woman from behind, especially if she is kneeling in front of him so she is at an angle with her bottom higher than her head, it is said to encourage conception – back strength permitting.

DOUBLE SPOONS

Making love in the spoons position (both partners lying cuddled into each other facing the same way, with the man penetrating the woman from behind) is not thought to be such an effective baby-making position because the penetration angle is not so deep. However, the chances can be maximized if the woman leans the upper half of her body a little

WHEN TO CURB YOUR URGE

Traditional Chinese medical texts say that there are nine conception times that may produce an unhealthy child and so should be avoided:

- Noon
- Midnight
- During a solar eclipse
- During a thunder or lightning storm
- During a rainbow
- During a summer or winter solstice (21 December or 21 June)
- At full moon

All the above are when the environment is highly polarized with electrical charges, or changing balance. The Chinese used to believe this could lead to a corresponding imbalance in the child's constitution. Other times to avoid are when either partner is drunk or full of food.

away from her partner while sensuously arching her back as much as is comfortable, bracing her hands against the wall or bed surface for extra purchase, and pushing her bottom against him.

POST-COITAL POSSUM

Some clinicians reckon that a woman is more likely to conceive if she lies still for up to half an hour after lovemaking, preferably with her legs up against the wall or with a pillow under her hips.

They suggest that, if she moves, the ejaculate fluid containing sperm is more likely to trickle out of her, and that the earth's gravitational pull will work against the sperm which remain inside and are trying to swim for the egg. They cite the fact that some female animals remain still for a while after intercourse for this reason. In addition, women naturally tend to feel sleepier than men after intercourse and are more inclined to want to have a nap, whilst men are more likely to want to get up and do something else after a few minutes' rest. This is thought to be nature's way of keeping women still in order to maximize their chances of successful conception.

However, this is all probably a bit unnecessary and potentially a source of additional stress (which couples may be feeling anyway if they are trying to get pregnant and it is taking longer than they thought). Studies show that the first – and therefore best and fittest – sperm have reached your Fallopian tubes in five minutes flat and even the laggards have usually got there within 45 minutes. So, as long as you don't leap up the moment you've finished every time, it is doubtful you really need to suffer the indignity and inconvenience of being stuck on the bed or the floor in a vulnerable position, with one eye on the clock.

In any case, it's the fastest and best sperm you want to fertilize your egg because they are more likely than the weaker latecomers to help your egg develop into a healthy embryo and stable pregnancy. As Dr Steve Brody of the Advanced Fertility Institute of San Diego puts it: 'The sperm that get in right away have the most chance of fertilizing the egg. A study in rabbits shows that if you destroy all sperm in the vagina within five minutes the rabbit will still become pregnant.' OK, so the human reproductive system is not the same as a rabbit's, but the point is a reasonable one.

Does it matter who is on top?

If the 'worst' conception positions include your personal favourites, don't take it too seriously. The truth is, as family planning doctor Dr Karen Trewinnard puts it: 'The best way to get pregnant is to have plenty of sex' – in any position. And it is important to enjoy it, because the best sex positions for you to conceive in are probably the ones you like best because you will be more relaxed. So take the advice above with a large pinch of salt, and, even if you suspect there may be something in the gravity story, remember that a female orgasm would probably counteract it and sperm are very energetic.

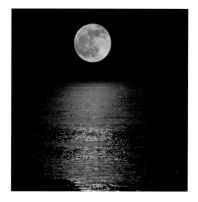

ABOVE The full moon is associated with fertility in many cultures and legends, although different countries disagree about its significance. The Chinese believe it is not a lucky time to make a baby, but Westerners feel that it is a time of rising sexuality and excitability for many living creatures – including humans.

'WORST' SEX POSITIONS FOR CONCEPTION

Supposedly, any position which goes against gravity and so discourages the sperm's upward joinery is thought to deter conception. They include:

- Woman on top
- Having sex sitting
- Having sex standing up

Sex selection positions

LOVEMAKING TO CREATE A BABY BOY

There is no evidence whatsoever for any of the following. However, folklore claims that if you want a boy you should:

- Stay lying down for half an hour after sex
- Make sure the woman sleeps on her partner's left after lovemaking
- Make love standing up
- Make love when there is a quarter moon in the sky
- Have sex at night
- Make love with the woman's head pointing north
- Have sex in the rear-entry position
- Make sure the man is the one to initiate sex
- Make sure the man climaxes first.

LOVEMAKING TO CREATE A BABY GIRL

Again, there is no evidence for the following, but the story goes that if you want a baby girl you should:

- Make love when the moon is full. At this time the moon is at its furthest from the sun so the ionosphere (upper atmosphere) is 'squeezed' towards earth. According to Dr Roger Coghill of Coghill Laboratories in Wales, this creates more positive ions in the air.

  Dr Coghill has studied the effect of electromagnetic fields on living things for the last 20 years, and has written about the established links between full moon and increased aggression, flare-ups in existing mental health conditions and general excitability. He also suggests a full moon can make the blood 'stickier', slowing down the circulation and reducing the blood's oxygen levels, which may produce more psychological stress. Stockbreeders know that the full moon affects the fertility of animals – but the sex ratio of babies? Who knows. However, if it increases excitability in living creatures, it could be a powerful time to have 'successful' sex anyway.
- Make love in mid-afternoon. Human testosterone levels which power sex drive are at their lowest at that time in both men and women, and at their highest at around 6am. The idea behind this one may be: less background testosterone (predominantly a male sex hormone), less chance of a boy.
- Make love on the 'even' days of the month. No one knows where this one comes from.
- Try a traditional Chinese conception chart. This is based on how old you are, what month you were born in and which month it is when you try to conceive.

It is also said that if the woman is the dominant one in the relationship at the time of conception she is more likely to have a girl.

Boy or Girl? Your Chance to Choose

There are certain methods used by doctors and parents that can, it seems, increase the likelihood of your having a daughter or a son. But here is how natural gender selection works when it is left to its own devices.

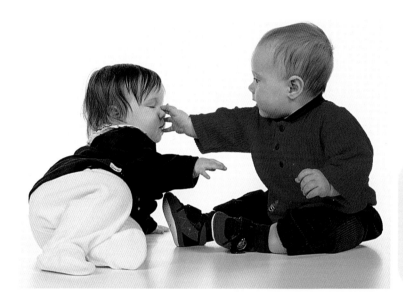

LEFT Couples are becoming ever more interested in trying to choose the sex of their future baby. But perhaps one question to ask first might be: 'Would we love and welcome the baby just as much if it wasn't the 'right' gender?'

DID YOU KNOW?
For the first six weeks of its life in the womb, the tiny embryo has not yet become either one sex or the other anyway, but is still neuter.

What happens naturally

A normal female cell has 22 pairs of ordinary chromosomes plus a pair of X sex chromosomes (referred to as XX). These sex chromosomes drive the development of all the special female characteristics such as the womb, ovaries and breasts.

An ordinary male cell also contains 22 pairs of ordinary chromosomes, plus a pair of sex chromosomes. This time, however, only one is an X, and the other is a Y, making the cell XY. It is the Y part that is responsible for developing all the male characteristics, such as the penis and testicles.

Sperm and egg cells are different from any other cells. Instead of the usual package of 46 chromosomes (23 pairs) they have just 23 chromosomes, one of which is the sex chromosome. In the case of the egg the sex chromosome will always be an X but in the sperm it will be either an X or a Y.

THE BIOLOGICAL BASIS OF CHOOSING YOUR BABY'S SEX

If it is an X-carrying sperm that meets the fertilized egg first, the baby will be a girl. If a Y-carrying sperm fertilizes the egg, the baby will be a boy. The theory of deliberate gender selection is based on enabling X sperm to get there first if the couple want a girl, or a Y sperm if the couple want a boy.

NEW DEVELOPMENTS
Researchers at the Genetics and IVF Institute in Fairfax, Vancouver, Canada, say they can help parents choose their baby's sex through a procedure called flow cytometry, in which DNA is stained with fluorescent dye and sorted.
However, the medical ethics aspects of this are still being hotly debated, unless the couple are trying to avoid specific inherited, sex-linked conditions such as haemophilia.

There are many superstitions about how to maximize your chances of having either a baby boy or a baby girl. Couples have been trying to influence the odds ever since the creation of inherited wealth.

The Ancient Greeks, for example, believed that one testicle contained the seed for producing girls and the other contained seed for boys, so they used to tie off one side with a linen or leather strip before making love. Some French noblemen, with their estates to think of and desperate for a male heir, went one step further and had a testicle amputated (there was no anaesthetic in those days either). In the Palau Islands of the Pacific the wife still dresses up in her husband's clothes before lovemaking if they are planning for a boy. Some traditional Austrian midwives still bury the placenta under a nut tree after the birth if asked to do so; this is supposed to increase the chances of the couple having a son next time around.

Since the 1970s, however, doctors have been becoming a bit more scientific about the art of gender pre-selection. Most methods are based on two fairly logical theories, but neither of them have yet been rigorously scientifically proven to the satisfaction of the general medical establishment, which still regards the subject with a professionally jaundiced eye.

THE GO-FASTER THEORY

This was initially proposed by Dr Sophie Kleegman, an infertility specialist practising in New York in the 1950s. She noticed that her artificial-insemination patients tended to have more girls, or more boys, depending on what day of the woman's menstrual cycle she had her treatment on. She concluded that this was happening because 'male' Y-carrying sperm swim faster but 'female' X-carrying sperm live longer.

Although Kleegman's theories were confirmed by later studies, it is only fair to mention that other scientists, such as Dr William James at London's University College, have found the exact opposite when they investigated the matter.

ACID VERSUS ALKALINE

The other theory is that male-producing Y sperm seem to prefer the naturally acidic environment of the woman's vagina and can survive there better than 'female' X sperm.

APPLYING THE THEORIES

So, for males it is 'faster and acidic', for females it is 'slower and alkaline'. All the doctors needed to do to make a good deal of money was to work out a straightforward way of applying the sex ratio rules. What they came up with was the following:

1 Time lovemaking either to catch the faster male sperm or to wait for the slower female sperm.
2 Make the woman's vagina either more acidic or more alkaline than usual. This will be friendlier to either male- or female-carrying

sperm. Douching was tried, but that seemed to kill far too many sperm of both persuasions. There was also a small possibility of infection – and local irritation if the mixture was too strong.

3 Separate out 'male' from 'female' sperm and use artificial insemination with the separated sperm. One method of separation involves using a centrifuge; because 'male' Y-bearing sperm are lighter they end up at the top, whereas the heavier X chromosome-bearing sperm are spun to the bottom. Another method, patented by Dr Roland Ericsson, tries to separate the boy/girl chromosome-bearing sperm by filtering them.

Remember, there are no guarantees, and some of the methods' rationales contradict each other. As Dr Weinberg of the National Institute of Environmental Health Sciences, USA, puts it: 'You can find a small study to support any theory.'

Dr Papa

In the mid-1980s, the aptly named Dr François Papa, a French obstetrician, came up with a more user-friendly approach involving diet. According to Dr Papa, a woman should eat foods rich in sodium and potassium if she wants a girl and one high in calcium and magnesium if she wants a boy. An 80+% success rate was claimed.

Many people still follow Dr Papa's suggestions. Here is what to eat:

Boy food
Eat: meat, tea, coffee, rice, pasta, alcohol, plenty of salty foods, fish, milk-free puddings and sauces, cornflakes, white breads, all fresh fruits, prunes, raisins, dates, figs, sugar, milk-free margarine, and all vegetables except those on the 'girl food' list.

Avoid: any form of milk, such as cheese and yogurts, pastries, shellfish, brown bread, salad vegetables, chocolate and nuts.

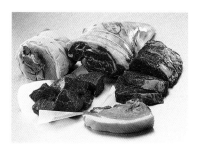

ABOVE If you are hoping for a boy baby, Dr Papa recommends plenty of red meat in your diet.

LEFT Good news for chocolate lovers who would like to have a baby girl – it's on the 'girl food' list to eat every day.

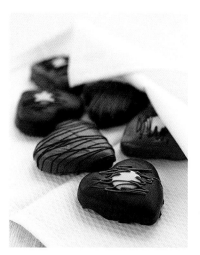

Girl food
Eat: dairy products such as milk puddings and unsalted cheeses/butter, yogurt, eggs; plenty of sweet foods such as jam, honey and chocolate every day; rice, semolina, pasta, foods containing cornflour, unsalted nuts, carrots, beans, turnips, onions, leeks, peas, peppers and cucumbers.

Avoid: salty foods, and salt added to food (read packaged food labels carefully to check for it).

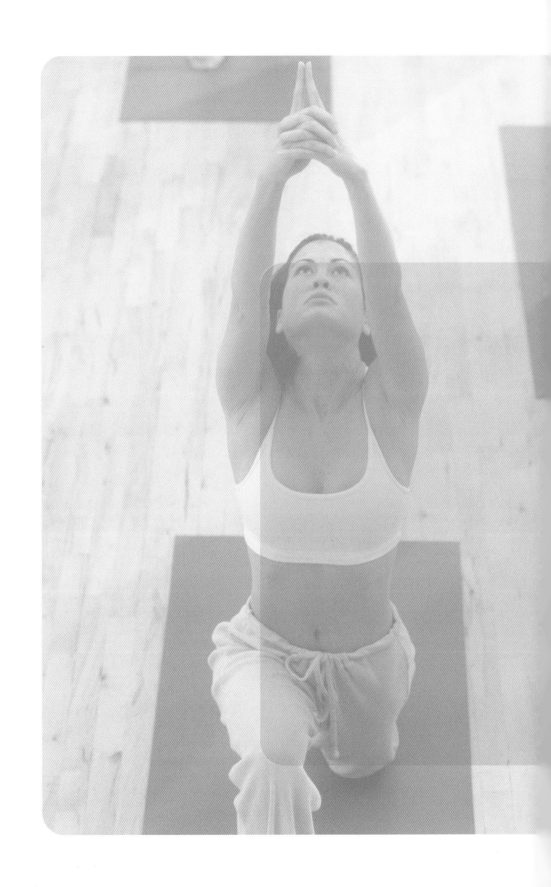

Self-help and Preconceptual Care

The rumours are true - there is more to becoming pregnant than having sex. Almost everything you do in the four short months leading up to trying for a baby can be as important as the sex itself. What you eat, drink, smoke, breathe, do as a job, how stressed you are, whether you are short of certain vital minerals or vitamins, what's in your physical environment, your emotional health - it all matters. Any one of them can make all the difference between you becoming pregnant and having a healthy baby, and not, especially if you are taking longer than you'd thought to conceive, or are having problems doing so.

Becoming as healthy as possible before you begin trying for a baby, to maximize your chances of success, is called preconceptual care. This is what the next section of the book is about. The good news is that most of the things are under your own control. Even better news is that this approach has helped many thousands of other couples to become pregnant and have healthy babies over the past 20 years.

Who says it works? There has been some groundbreaking research by Surrey University in the UK looking at 367 couples who were trying to conceive, over a period of three years. The women were aged 22-45, the men 25-59. Nearly four out of ten had a history of infertility. The same number of couples had suffered up to five miscarriages each. Many, especially the older men and women, had come to the trial as a last resort. By the end of the trial, nine out of ten of these couples had given birth to healthy babies. Even 65% of those who had tried IVF without success became pregnant without any further treatments.

It worked for them. It could work for you, too.

What is Preconceptual Care and Why Does it Make a Difference?

A good preconceptual care programme can help you to:

- **get pregnant more quickly**
- **minimize the risk of a miscarriage**
- **maximize your chances of creating a baby who is well and healthy.**

Preconceptual care involves getting both partners into the best possible physical and mental shape to maximize your chances of creating a pregnancy that lasts to full term, and brings you a healthy baby at the end of it. A three- to four-month programme of healthy living will get you into good shape before trying for a baby. Research suggests that if you do this you are likely to become pregnant more quickly and to have less chance of miscarriage.

What do I have to do?

There is no magic formula – most of it is common sense. Yet, for couples who are experiencing difficulty in becoming pregnant, the results of doing all the five steps to fertility together (rather than maybe just one or two) can be dramatic (see box left).

Who says it works?

Many research studies (see References, page 136) have suggested that a shortage of certain vitamins and minerals can reduce sperm quality and count, as can smoking and alcohol. It is well known that smoking can damage eggs, and that even small amounts of toxic substances from ordinary household and work sources can reduce your fertility.

Over the last 25 years a British organization called Foresight has pioneered an approach to human fertility that takes into account diet, exposure to pollutants, infections and nutritional status, which seems to give a remarkably high success (live baby) rate of 80%. Independent research by Surrey University confirms that Foresight's method is indeed effective. For three years the university team followed the fortunes of 367 couples who had had difficulties in becoming pregnant or having a healthy baby. The couples were instructed to follow a regime which involved detoxing, being tested for mineral and vitamin shortages and having these put right with supplements and by eating organic food. Any infections were treated. By the end of three years, nine out of ten of the couples had a healthy baby.

It is interesting to note that some of these couples had previously tried *in-vitro* fertilization (IVF) without success, and of these couples, 65% conceived naturally on the Foresight regime.

FIVE STEPS TO FERTILITY
For at least four months before trying for a baby, both partners should:

1 Eat only healthy, fresh foods.
2 Eliminate any toxic substances from your system – for instance, give up smoking and drinking alcohol.
3 Find out which minerals, vitamins or other nutrients you are short of, and top up.
4 Become as fit and well as you can be (for example exercise regularly; get checked for and treat low-level genito-urinary infections such as thrush).
5 Reduce the level of stress in your life wherever you possibly can.

Not one of the women miscarried either. The usual average rate for confirmed pregnancies is one in seven, so in 367 couples you would usually expect there to be around 50.

How does preconceptual care work?

What you take into your body helps to form the building blocks for the makeup of every single cell, including sperm and eggs. The healthier you are as a whole, the healthier your eggs or sperm and the better your chances of conceiving sooner rather than later, and of the pregnancy going on to give you a healthy baby at the end of it.

Why do both partners need to follow a pre-pregnancy programme?

Granted, it's the woman who grows the baby inside her and nourishes it with her body's resources. But it takes one special cell from *each* partner – a sperm from him and an egg from her – to make a child. If either of you are less than healthy, you may have difficulty getting pregnant in the first place, and you are more likely to miscarry.

WHY PREPARE FOR FOUR MONTHS?
It takes three months to make a new batch of sperm cells from scratch. It also takes between six weeks and three months to eliminate certain toxins from your system properly and to raise the level of certain vital nutrients in your blood serum.

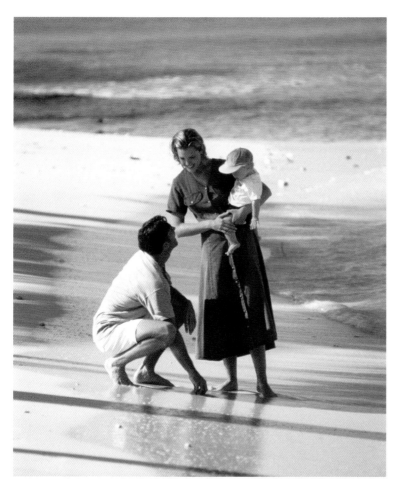

LEFT If both partners are physically and emotionally well, research suggests they stand a far better chance of conceiving more quickly, avoiding miscarriage and having a good pregnancy resulting in a healthy, full-term baby.

Preconceptual Care for Women

If you decide that you are ready to try for a baby, your first move should be to go to your doctor for a general check-up. This needs to include the following:

- **Blood pressure check**.
- **Urine test for infection**, and also for **glucose**. Up to 1 in 20 women is predisposed to diabetes and can temporally develop it in pregnancy. This is called gestational diabetes, and it means a close check has to be kept on their blood-sugar levels, or there are potential health problems for both them and their baby.
- **A cervical smear** to ensure your cervix is healthy.
- **A blood-group test** to see if you are Rhesus negative.
- **A discussion of any long-term health conditions**, such as diabetes, early-onset arthritis, multiple sclerosis (MS), HIV (human immunodeficiency virus) infection, and their implications for pregnancy and motherhood.
- **A check on your immune status**, especially for rubella (German measles) and toxoplasmosis. You need to be vaccinated for rubella at least three months before you begin trying for a baby.
- **An investigation for silent genito-urinary infections** that could affect either your chances of becoming pregnant or the pregnancy itself. (You can go to your local genito-urinary clinic for this if you prefer.) Nearly three-quarters of all women are thought to be infected with chlamydia, for example. In most cases this is mild without any symptoms at all; however, it can sometimes cause infertility or subfertility, miscarriage and ectopic pregnancy.
- **A discussion of any medication you are taking**. Check with your doctor that it is definitely safe to take it in pregnancy and that it will not affect your fertility. Certain drugs used to control epilepsy, for example, carry a raised risk of birth defects, so you may need to change to a prescription that is safer. See Drugs and medicines, page 71.

TRANQUILLIZERS AND SLEEPING PILLS

Few people go through life without needing these at some point, even if only for root canal work at the dentist. About 13 million prescriptions for some form of anti-anxiety drugs or treatments for insomnia are given in the UK every year. You probably already know that tranquillizers are addictive – most are only recommended for short-term courses of about six weeks. What you may not know is that they can also affect your unborn baby (see Benzo babies, page 73).

If you have been prescribed tranquillizers, try the very best you can to quit them before you become pregnant. If your doctor does not offer you full support to come off them slowly, there are organizations that can advise and support you, as this type of medication can be notoriously difficult to give up (see Helplines, page 139).

Body weight matters

One thing that gives you a flying start in the getting-pregnant stakes is being around the right weight. The first bit of reasonable news (since 27% women and men in Britain are currently dieting, and 40% of women are 'being careful what they eat') is that the ideal weight for conceiving is heavier than you would think.

For a woman of average height – say 162 cm (5 ft 4 inches), medium frame – the optimum *fertility* weight, that is the ideal weight range for becoming pregnant, is about 55–66 kg (122–145 lb) though your optimum weight for *general* health is lower – between 50 and 63 kg (110–139 lb). If you are 168 cm (5 ft 6 inches) tall your optimum fertility

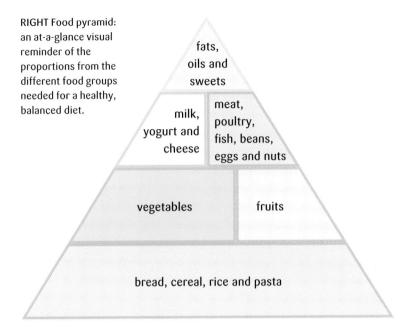

RIGHT Food pyramid: an at-a-glance visual reminder of the proportions from the different food groups needed for a healthy, balanced diet.

fats, oils and sweets

milk, yogurt and cheese

meat, poultry, fish, beans, eggs and nuts

vegetables

fruits

bread, cereal, rice and pasta

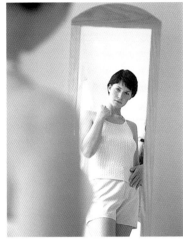

ABOVE Being underweight (by only 5 kg/10 lbs or so) is one of the most common reasons for otherwise healthy women finding it hard to conceive.

weight is around 59–71 kg (131–157 lb) and your optimum general health weight is 53–67 kg (117–147 lb).

UNDERWEIGHT?

Media images tell us that a sexy body is a very slim body, but the skinny catwalk model shape is not what a healthy woman looks like. It may look good in clothes, but dieting for weight loss affects your output of hormones, which can stop your ovaries ripening and releasing eggs. It may also make your periods erratic, sometimes stopping them altogether.

FAT IS ESSENTIAL TO FERTILITY

A certain percentage of body fat is vital for fertility. Women are supposed to be fatter than men for a very good reason – we need it to ovulate. Young girls do not begin their periods until they have at least 17% body fat. The average woman has 27% of her weight as body fat.

However, you can have too much of a good thing. Statistics for 2001 from the UK's National Audit Office show that over half of all British women are either overweight or clinically obese. And being overweight can stop you ovulating. This may be because the extra fat produces a little extra oestrogen in your system, causing an imbalance in the ratio of the reproductive hormones needed for egg ripening and release.

However, the effect is quickly and easily reversed. One piece of research in 1998 showed that just losing a small amount of weight, such as 10%, can be enough to stimulate ovulation again and make periods more regular. In another small study by the University of Adelaide in 1995 involving 12 overweight women who were not ovulating, after following a six-month programme of steady exercise and diet, 11 of them conceived naturally.

SAFE, EASIER WEIGHT LOSS

- Aim to lose just 1 kg (2 lb) a week. It may not sound much but it soon adds up.
- Don't crash diet. Much of what you'll lose is water, and it'll come straight back on again as soon as you begin to eat normally anyway.
- Exercise three times a week or more.
- If you are using a hormonal form of contraception, check with your family planning clinic or doctor that it is not making you put on weight.
- Get checked out for food intolerances, allergies and candida, all of which can cause bloating, water retention and weight gain.
- Cut calories by limiting your intake of fatty foods. Go for skimmed and half-fat options instead.
- Eat plenty of fresh fruit and vegetables.

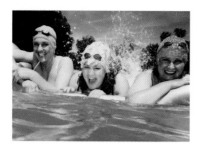

ABOVE If you pick a form of exercise you really enjoy and that is actually fun or satisfying to you, you will find that your new exercise regime lasts far longer than the most ferocious personal training programme.

Exercise can improve your fertility

You don't have to be fit to be fertile but it helps. If you are reasonably physically fit this increases your chances of conceiving quickly, and it will also help you have a more comfortable pregnancy and easier birth. Exercise also reduces stress, promotes good sleep patterns, improves your circulation, breathing systems and stamina levels, and improves your feeling of both physical and mental wellbeing. And when you are feeling this good your confidence and sex drive bloom.

Exercising regularly also:

- improves the blood supply to your reproductive organs
- can regulate your menstrual cycle by helping you reach a healthy body weight, and keeping stress levels down
- encourages you to increase your natural mineral, vitamin and other positive nutrient intake by stimulating your appetite without allowing you to gain weight.

THE EASIER WAY TO EXERCISE

It is much easier to fit exercise into your life if you pick an activity you can do conveniently and easily, and also something you actually like doing. Check out the logistics of your fitness options.

For instance, swimming is a good idea if you have a pool within easy reach of home or work, but not if the only one is miles out of your way. Running in the park during your lunch hour is a great idea as long as you do not have to be back at work immediately after lunch looking immaculate every day. The same applies to cycling to work, unless there are decent washroom facilities and somewhere to strip off any sweaty cycling gear. A step aerobics class or squash is all very well after a long, stressful day at work if you've got enough energy left. If you haven't, then try something more calming and less frenetic. Belly-dancing? T'ai Chi? Martial arts?

HOW FIT ARE YOU RIGHT NOW?

Test yourself:
- Can you walk briskly for 15 minutes without getting puffed out?
- Sit down quietly, and check your resting pulse rate. Feel for it where your wrist joins your hand, just below your thumb and about 1 cm (½ inch) from the wrist-edge. Count the beats for 15 seconds, then multiply by 4. If the result is under 70, you are pretty fit; 80–100, not too bad, but not great. Over 100 – you are not in good physical health.

What's your poison? Cigarettes and alcohol for women

Purist preconceptual advisors insist that even one alcoholic drink (just a little one) or a single cigarette could be damaging if you drink it or smoke it at a crucial time for egg development. Are they being unreasonably strict - or could they be right?

CIGARETTES

Certainly a woman can become pregnant if she smokes cigarettes, and many women do. However, it can make things far harder for many and downright impossible for some - which is why research shows that women who do not smoke are twice as likely to become pregnant within a year of trying as women who do.

Cigarettes reduce oestrogen levels. Specialists think that this may be because the granulosa cells, which make oestrogen and surround each unripe egg, are inhibited by the toxins from cigarettes. If there is not enough oestrogen in your system, the body will not make enough luteinizing hormone (LH); and, because this is the hormone that stimulates an egg to ripen each month, the result will be that no egg is released.

Lowered oestrogen levels:

UP IN SMOKE
Smoking can bring on an earlier menopause, which may be relevant for a woman who is in her late thirties or early forties and trying for a baby. The fertility of a 35-year-old woman who smokes an average of 5–10 cigarettes a day is the same as that of a 40-year-old non-smoker.

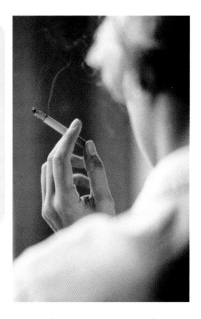

ABOVE If you are a woman smoker you can increase your chances of becoming pregnant from the moment you give up, or significantly cut down on, cigarettes.

- cut down the number of fertile years you have left to conceive a baby, and bring your menopause closer
- cause irregular periods
- make your eggs more impenetrable to sperm
- affect the consistency of your cervical mucus, making it more difficult for sperm to swim through.

If you are a smoker and you quit, your fertility and chances of a healthy baby begin to improve right away. Even if you are newly pregnant, it's not too late to stop and do some good. However, since the effects of smoking take a few months to recede properly, try to stop at least four to six months before you begin trying for a baby. This is probably one of the most important things you can do for your preconceptual care. If you feel you could do with some support or practical advice, call a support group or talk to your doctor. Reflexology, acupuncture, hypnotherapy or Autogenic Training may all help support you as you attempt to give up smoking.

ALCOHOL

Drinking alcohol may reduce your fertility too, and a study in the *British Medical Journal* in 1998 states categorically that women 'should be warned to avoid alcohol when trying to conceive'.

Heavy drinking can sometimes prevent ovulation altogether, but that is not usual. The problem is more likely to be that alcohol may prevent enough progesterone being produced by the egg capsule (corpus luteum) in the ovary in the very early part of pregnancy. This would inhibit implantation of the fertilized egg in the womb lining or would cause it to lose its hold. Progesterone is one of the major players in ensuring a pregnancy stays put. One survey of 32,000 women in Jerusalem in 1980 found that women who drank as little as 1–2 units of alcohol a day were twice as likely to miscarry as women who did not drink any alcohol at all.

Bug-busting

There are a number of genito-urinary (GU) infections (affecting the water works and genitals) that can either stop you getting pregnant or cause miscarriages. You may not even know that you have one, as many people have no noticeable symptoms.

It is very important indeed that both partners have a broad, blanket screening for GU infections before you even begin trying for a baby, especially if the woman has had a miscarriage before. Probably the best place to have this done is a specialist GU clinic. You do not need a doctor's referral to go to one and all results are treated in complete confidence so they will not even inform your own doctor if you don't want them to do so. GU clinics treat everything from ordinary thrush to venereal disease and from genital warts to herpes.

CHLAMYDIA

The Royal College of Physicians estimates this is the most common sexually transmitted disease of them all. Often symptomless in men and women, up to 70% of women who have it don't realize that they do. Chlamydia may cause full-blown infertility in women because the inflammation may scar and block the Fallopian tubes down which a ripe egg needs to travel to meet the sperm. It can also cause inflammation of the cervix, which can result in temporary infertility by affecting the cervical mucus.

DOUBLE CHECK
Tests for chlamydia are not 100% accurate. If one partner tests positive for the infection, is essential that *both* of you are treated, even if the other partner's test says they are clear.

If you have a chlamydia infection and are already pregnant it is important to treat it right away as it can be passed on to your baby, possibly causing severe eye and lung infections. If caught early, it can be successfully treated with antibiotics.

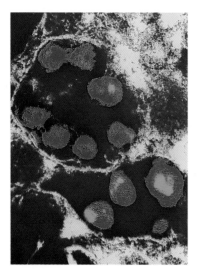

ABOVE Close up of just one of the bugs which can play havoc with your fertility.

TRICHOMONIASIS

In women this infection causes an unpleasant greenish discharge and sore vagina and vulva; men may experience a sore penis tip and inflammation of the urethra. Trichomoniasis will not cause pelvic infection as chlamydia can, but it may reduce fertility by changing the quality of a woman's cervical mucus, making it more difficult (or impossible) for sperm to swim through. A course of antibiotics should clear it up.

MYCOPLASMA AND UREAPLASMA

These organisms are commonly found in the GU tracts of both men and women but more are found in couples who are having difficulty becoming pregnant. Research suggests that mycoplasma may increase the percentage of abnormal sperm and may affect sperm by lowering the amount of zinc and fructose in semen. Zinc is important for sperm and fructose is the sugar that the sperm use as fuel for their journey up through the vagina and womb to the egg.

Research that was published in America in 1983 also linked these microbes with miscarriage, so if you have previously had an unexplained miscarriage it may be well worth getting yourself screened for mycoplasma or ureaplasma.

HIV

In 2001 there were 30,000 HIV-positive people in England and Wales, and it is estimated that about one in every three of them does not realize it. This may be one reason why some women decide to have a peace-of-mind HIV test before they begin trying for a baby.

A couple's actual fertility may not be affected by being HIV-positive, and someone with HIV infection may remain well for quite a long time – between six and 15 years, sometimes longer. When they do begin to experience symptoms of AIDS-related illnesses there are powerful drug cocktails available that can help to support them for a variable number of years more. However, there is, at the moment, no cure for AIDS.

If a mother has HIV, her baby acquires her antibodies through the placenta. Antibodies do not necessarily mean infection, though, and if the child is *not* infected these antibodies will disappear by the time he or she is about 18 months old.

In England and Wales (at the time of writing in 2001) there have been reports of about 1,600 babies born to HIV-positive mothers. Of these, 38% of the babies were infected, 40% were shown not to be, and for the rest no one is yet sure. A mother who is pregnant and HIV-positive can take certain preventative measures during pregnancy, birth and her baby's infancy which, according to the UK Public Health Laboratory Service, can 'almost eliminate' the risk of her child being infected too. The main ones are taking antiviral drug treatment in the last trimester of her pregnancy, having a special 'bloodless' caesarean birth using laser surgery, and bottle-feeding her baby rather than breast-feeding.

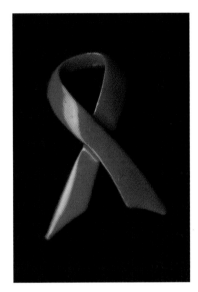

ABOVE Many women are now choosing to have an HIV peace-of-mind test before they are pregnant or in the early stages of pregnancy since, though it may not affect your ability to conceive, the infection may have major implications for your parenthood.

CMV (CYTOMEGALOVIRUS)

This is a member of the family of herpes viruses, and while infection should not make any difference to a woman's fertility it may affect the man's by reducing his sperm count. CMV has also been linked to an increased risk of miscarriage, and has been associated with a range of problems, including eye infections, hearing loss and brain damage, for unborn babies if they contract it in the womb via their mother.

Emotional Health

Good emotional health involves not just the absence of problems and disorders, but a positive state in which everything is in reasonable balance. When asked to describe it, psychologists include the following as signs of a good state: feeling (at least) reasonably happy; having pretty stable moods which are not on a constant roller coaster; being able to connect with others; being able to give and receive affection or love freely; feeling emotions fully and reacting to them appropriately; being able to gain enjoyment and satisfaction from your personal relationships, both at home and at work, and sensual pleasure from sex, food and drink.

Like good physical health, emotional health is important for fertility, conception and pregnancy. People can certainly conceive if they are in emotional distress or upheaval, but for many it proves more difficult (see Stress and infertility, page 59). Bodies have in-built mechanisms which can prevent you from becoming pregnant (or getting your partner pregnant) at times when we do not feel secure, or when we are simply not yet ready for it. If there are areas of difficulty or strain in your life these may be harder to cope with, or put right, when you are pregnant, or have a small baby to care for.

It can be easier to spot emotional strain or imbalance in others rather than in ourselves because living with a constant state of, say, anxiety, can start to feel almost normal (or at least, usual), especially if it has crept up on you gradually.

The questions below are just a very limited guide, but may perhaps start you thinking 'How am I really feeling?' Instead of automatically answering 'OK' (the response most people expect to have to make if someone asks them how they are), perhaps some of the questions may strike a chord with you or help indicate areas of stress, or distress, in your life that would be better if they were tackled or talked about.

The talk could be with a lover, a good friend, a parent, or a professional counsellor. Counsellors are primarily guiding sounding-boards. A good one will not tell you what you are feeling or what to do. Instead, they are trained to listen, to support, and to help us identify those parts of life that may not be doing us as much good as we would like. Then, and only then, might they start helping you to explore what you would like to do about those areas.

HOW ARE YOU FEELING AT THE MOMENT?

1 Do you ever get angry, sound off at someone and think: heavens, where did that come from?
(a) Frequently (b) Occasionally
(c) Seldom

2 Would you describe your moods as
(a) Pretty even (b) Erratic pre-menstrually (c) Quite volatile?

3 Do you laugh out loud at least once a day?
(a) Yes (b) No

4 If you are annoyed or angry with someone do you find it easy to tell them?
(a) Yes (b) No, I bottle it up
(c) It takes me a while

5 Do you ever catch yourself feeling happy or contented for no particular reason?
(a) Frequently (b) Sometimes
(c) There needs to be a good reason

6 Would you say you get enjoyment and pleasure from food and drink?
(a) Usually, unless I am in a rush
(b) I regard it more as fuel (c) Not really. I eat because I know I should

7 Do you wake feeling alert and refreshed after a night's sleep?
(a) Yes (b) Reasonably (c) No, I often wake still feeling tired

8 Do you ever find yourself drinking more than you know you should?
(a) Very occasionally (b) Sometimes
(c) Often

9 Do you ever wake up already feeling anxious?
(a) No (b) Occasionally
(c) Frequently

10 Take a moment to check how you are breathing right this minute.
(a) Are you taking deep, regular

breaths? (b) Do you seem to be breathing only half way down into your chest? (c) Have you just caught yourself holding your breath – again?

11 If you have a lot of urgent work to get through this morning or several difficult phone calls to make, would you be

(a) Quite looking forward to getting it out of the way (b) Resigned: let's get on with it (c) Stressed, uncertain where to begin (d) Fiddling about to avoid getting started?

12 How would you describe your sex drive at the moment?

(a) Same, or higher than, usual (b) Average (c) Not that interested, though feel you should be (d) Too tired at the moment to feel sexy

13 Do you like socializing and seeing friends at the moment?

(a) Yes, as much as ever (b) Yes, but can't do as much as I'd like these days (c) No, I don't seem to have the emotional energy for it right now

14 Do you find it easy at the moment to allow yourself to feel strong emotions like happiness, sympathy, and enthusiasm?

(a) Yes (b) Sometimes (c) No, it has to be something really major

15 Do you like your own body – are you happy to be inhabiting it?

(a) Yes, pretty much (b) There are some things I wish I could change (c) Not much (d) I often feel angry with it/annoyed with it for letting me down/dislike it

16 If someone criticizes you heavily out of the blue, would you tend to

(a) Be taken aback, but later wonder if maybe you could learn something (b) Go away and think about it (c) Feel upset and insecure (d) Be furious and defend yourself angrily?

17 Do you find it very frustrating when other people will not fall in with things you have carefully planned?

(a) No, it's their loss (b) It's a bit disappointing (c) It makes me see red when I have taken the trouble to organize something

18 If you have had a brief row with someone or they have wronged you in some fairly small way, do you find it easy to let it go afterwards?

(a) Yes (b) Can take a while (c) No, I can sulk for days

19 Do you have any interests, enthusiasms or hobbies outside work or home?

(a) One or two (b) They seem to be taking over my life (c) Would quite like to but cannot seem to find the time (d) Can't seem to find anything I fancy

20 Would you say the amount of stress in your life is currently

(a) Less than usual (b) About the same – average (c) About the same – too much (d) Worse than usual?

21 Does the prospect of major change - say moving house, a new job, choosing to downsize your life – make you feel

(a) Excited (b) A bit wary (c) Tired at the very thought (d) Nervous?

22 Do you feel in control of your life?

(a) More or less (b) Sometimes (c) Not right now (d) I wish I did

23 It's party time, you're tired and a group of friends are coming to stay. Are you

(a) Looking forward to it hugely (b) A bit anxious – that's a lot of people for you at the moment (c) Very anxious: how are you going to cope with all that (d) Resigned?

24 Do you find it easy and natural to express physical affection when you feel it?

(a) Sure (b) Yes, but I can feel a bit awkward (c) No

25 'If what you're doing isn't working, change what you're doing.' Does that strike you as

(a) Obvious, but brilliant when you think about it (b) Fortune cookie wisdom (c) I wouldn't know where to start (d) Stupid – nothing's that simple?

SCORING

Mostly a - Emotionally healthy. You are on an even keel, and your life is pretty balanced. You can feel and express a wide range of appropriate emotions, are probably interested in many aspects of life and the world around you, and know a thing or two about enjoying yourself.

Mostly b - Reasonably emotionally healthy. Yet perhaps you also need to slow down a bit and give yourself some extra latitude. Try to think about which things really are the most important to you and make sure you have room and time for them. Believe that what you want and feel matters.

Mostly c and d - Do you ever wake up in the morning and think: How did life get this way? Perhaps it's time to stop and take stock, to think about what you need from the different areas in your life - and perhaps talk it over with a good friend or counsellor to help clarify your thoughts or get some support.

Which Contraception?

If you have decided that you would like to have a child, contraception may be the last thing you'd think you would need to look at. Yet while you are preparing for pregnancy you may want to use a form of contraception that you can trust not to let you get pregnant before you are ready, but that will allow your fertility to return promptly when you stop using it.

Which are most effective?

Some of the most effective forms of contraception are hormonal methods, such as the combined pill, progestogen injections and progestogen implants. But these can also be the very ones that may delay the return of a woman's fertility.

THE COMBINED PILL

The combined pill is 99+% effective at preventing pregnancy. It works mainly by preventing ovulation. After stopping taking it, most women ovulate within six to eight weeks, some within as little as ten days. Women who have been using the triphasic pill, rather than a monophasic variety which has the same dose every day, may find that their fertility returns more quickly.

However, women over 30 may experience longer delays of up to a year (occasionally more), especially those who have not had any previous pregnancies.

THE PROGESTOGEN-ONLY PILL

The progestogen-only pill is also 99% effective, probably even more so for women over 35. It works by thickening the cervical mucus so that sperm cannot pass through into the womb. If you miss a single dose, fertility can return within 48 hours. There is no evidence of any delay in return of fertility after you stop using it.

THE IUD (INTRAUTERINE DEVICE)

The intrauterine device is 98–99% effective, depending on which one is used. It is a small plastic device with fine copper wire wound around it that works by causing a mild inflammation in the womb so its lining will not allow a fertilized egg to implant. An IUD will also inhibit the sperm's ability to move. Fertility usually returns promptly after an IUD's removal, unless it caused any pelvic infections while it was in place. If such an infection reaches the Fallopian tubes and causes scarring, the blockage this can produce may affect future fertility (see page 114).

THE IUS (INTRAUTERINE SYSTEM)

The intrauterine system is 99+% effective. This type of IUD has no copper wire, but instead is impregnated with progestogen. It releases a

NATURAL FAMILY PLANNING (NFP)

By learning to recognize the signals your body gives when you ovulate (that is your most fertile time of the month), you can work out when not to have intercourse and so avoid pregnancy. You can also use this the other way around, to work out the best time to make love if you want to get pregnant.

This technique is often encouraged by preconceptual care advisors. However, couples who are interested in using NFP to help them work out the best time to conceive really need to be in no special hurry to begin trying for a baby. It takes about three to six months to learn this method properly and to become confident and comfortable with it.

tiny amount of the hormone continuously, which acts directly on the womb's lining. The IUS prevents pregnancy by making the lining unwelcoming to a fertilized egg. It also inhibits sperm movement and thickens the cervical mucus guarding the entrance to the womb so that sperm can't swim through it. It may also inhibit, or partially prevent, ovulation.

Ovulation and periods usually begin again between one and two months after the removal of an IUS. If you are one of the 60% of women in whom it has not suppressed ovulation, your periods and fertility should return within a month. If it did suppress ovulation, fertility may take a bit longer, usually two months but occasionally more, to return.

CONTRACEPTIVE INJECTIONS
These are long-acting progestogen injections, such as Depo-Provera, which offer over 99% protection against pregnancy for 12 weeks. Another is called Noristerat and gives protection for eight weeks. These injections work by stopping ovulation, thickening the cervical mucus, and making your womb lining thinner and less likely to accept a fertilized egg. Your fertility and periods may take several months to return after stopping these injections. The average time is about six months, but a year is not uncommon and it may take up to 18 months, even if you have only ever had a single injection.

HORMONAL IMPLANTS
Implants are 98–99% effective, depending on which type is used. One type in common use is called Implanon. It is a single flexible rubber tube about the size of a hairgrip, which is placed underneath the skin of the inner upper arm. It releases a steady stream of progestogen into the bloodstream for three years, preventing ovulation. The manufacturers claim that after removal your fertility will return right away.

Another type, called Norplant, which consists of six small tubes, has recently been discontinued. However, some women still have these in place as they work for five years. Norplant prevents pregnancy by thickening the cervical mucus, making the lining of the womb thinner, and may also stop ovulation. After removal, you have a one in five chance of ovulating within a month, and most women will have done so by seven to eight weeks. Occasionally, fertility takes up to 18 months or more to return.

BARRIER METHODS
Barrier methods of contraception include the diaphragm, cervical cap, condoms and female condoms. If used with spermicides, these are between 95% and 98% effective. Barrier methods work by physically stopping sperm from reaching the small passageway that runs through the centre of the cervix. Spermicides work by killing sperm.

Your fertility will return as soon as you stop using any of these barrier methods, which makes them a popular choice for couples who want to delay pregnancy for just a few months longer while they follow a preconceptual care programme.

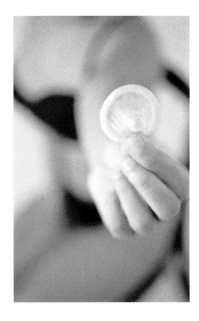

BELOW Because they contain no hormones, have no side-effects and are easy to use, sheaths are a popular choice as interim contraception for couples who are doing a three- to four-month preconceptual care programme before beginning to try for a baby.

Preconceptual Care for Men

It is thought that in 40% of couples with infertility problems the difficulty lies solely with the man, and a further 10-20% of the time both partners have some sort of fertility difficulty. For men, the most common reproductive problem is sperm *quality* - not just the sheer weight of numbers (it only takes one, in theory), but how many of them are swimming strongly and straight, what proportion is normally formed and whether they are able to penetrate a ripe egg when they reach one.

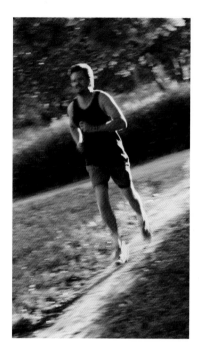

ABOVE Enthusiasm alert: a sudden burst of unaccustomed hefty exercise - like starting a keep-fit regime with a pair of expensive new Nikes and five-mile run every morning - can halve a man's sperm count. Take it gradually.

Both sperm quality and quantity can be substantially affected by many different lifestyle factors, ranging from too little or too much exercise, cigarette-smoking, street drug use and alcohol consumption, through to the wearing of tight underpants. This gives a man a substantial measure of control over his own fertility, and sperm have been shown to improve considerably in response to the most ordinary of DIY health measures. They do so pretty quickly too because sperm take only three months to mature and their production level could be the envy of any factory manager - most men are making 1,000 every second.

Exercise

Though most men's-health articles exhort them to start exercising regularly, recent American research suggests that if you suddenly launch into a major programme with all the enthusiasm of the newly converted, it can actually halve your sperm count. The study also shows that it may stay low for three months afterwards.

A sudden period of extra exercise also increases the number of immature, and therefore non-fertile, sperm found in semen. This may be because there is a natural fall in testosterone levels immediately after exercise. However, according to the National Sports Medicine Institute in the UK, regular, frequent players of sport are thought to have testosterone levels which are permanently slightly raised.

Exercise is excellent for de-stressing and overall fitness, but in order to maximize your fertility:

- keep to a sensible training regime - don't overdo it
- if you are starting a new sport or exercise programme to get yourself fitter, take it easy. Aim for three times a week. More isn't necessarily better.

Body weight

Many men in the Western world are overweight. In fact, nearly 40% of men in Britain weigh more than they should. If this includes you, it will affect your fertility because fat can cause circulating male hormones to break down into the female sex hormone oestrogen. The more over-weight you are, the more this will happen.

The most effective way to tackle excess poundage is (you've heard this one before) to take regular exercise two or three times a week, eat as healthily as possible and reduce your alcohol intake.

Alcohol

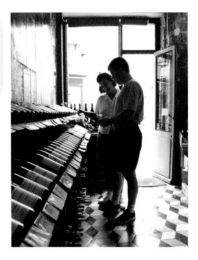

> **DID YOU KNOW?**
> Up to 40% of men's infertility problems have been blamed on alcohol.

Alcohol affects some men's fertility more than others. However, you can wipe out your sperm count for up to three months after a single heavy drinking session, according to Anthony Harsh, andrologist at Whipps Cross Hospital. This is because drinking alcohol reduces the level of vital sperm-making hormones (such as FSH and LH) sent out by the pituitary and hypothalamus gland, which causes sperm production to drop.

Men who drink four units of alcohol a day run a risk of lowered sperm count, and research by Dr Marsha Morgan at the Royal Free Hospital in London found that as little as one pint of beer (2 units) a day could produce abnormalities in semen. One unit is equivalent to half a pint of beer or lager, a glass of wine or a single shot of spirits.

The good news is that the effect can be quickly reversed. In Dr Morgan's study, men with low sperm counts were asked to avoid alcohol completely for three months. After a single month 40% of them were showing major improvements. Other research suggests that, if men with poor sperm counts or poor-quality sperm stop drinking, 50% will be back to normal within three months.

A constant intake of alcohol may also cause a man's system to produce a little extra oestrogen and less testosterone. This can have a slight feminizing effect on the body, such as male breast development, also known as gynaecomastia.

Preconceptual care experts insist that any man who wants to father a healthy child should stop drinking altogether for at least three months before trying to get his partner pregnant. This allows a new supply of alcohol-free sperm to develop.

For many people, a few drinks when you go out in the evenings are an enjoyable and, for some, pretty important part of social life. But look at it this way, it is only for a few months (perhaps as few as three) before you start trying for a baby. Then as soon as your partner becomes pregnant you can start to drink again if you want to.

ABOVE Good wine is one of life's great pleasures. Unfortunately men who drink 4+ units per day (two pints of beer or four glasses of wine) have lowered sperm count and half the sperm they do make are abnormal and won't move properly. Alcohol, especially beer, makes you put on weight. Obesity reduces testosterone production and sex drive in men and losing some weight increases it again.

> **DRUNKEN SPERM**
> Even if sperm production is not affected, alcohol can impair sperm's ability to reach the egg successfully - they appear to be simply too drunk to find their way up the Fallopian tubes.

Smoking cigarettes

Stopping smoking is, along with stopping booze, the other thing that fertility clinics strongly recommend prospective fathers to do. This is because the chemicals taken in while smoking, such as nicotine itself and carbon monoxide, increase the levels of damaging free radical

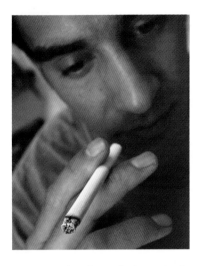

ABOVE Smokers have a higher ratio of abnormal sperm. If one of these does fertilize an egg, it brings with it a higher risk of that pregnancy miscarrying. Smokers' overall sperm counts are lower than non-smokers', too.

PATCH IT UP
Nicotine patches can be a useful stop-smoking aid. However, don't use patches or nicotine gum for four months before – or during – the time you and your partner are trying for a baby.

DID YOU KNOW?
Heat is so deadly for sperm production that a form of contraception based on 'tight underpants' has been developed and made available in France. It works by holding the testes so snugly against the body that they cannot stay cool enough to make sperm. The wearer's count dwindles to virtually zero. Unfortunately, the garment is so hot and uncomfortable that it is not a success.

molecules in the system, making cigarettes powerful antifertility agents. It has been shown that smoking can:

- Reduce your sperm count
- Affect your sperm's ability to move (motility)
- Cause impotence. Smoking can waste your ability to get, and sustain, an erection in the first place. Research by the British Medical Association and Action on Smoking and Health in 1999 estimated that one in ten (120,000) young British men in their thirties and forties have potency problems (difficulties keeping an erection up, 'soft' erections and total impotence) because they smoke, but this is something which never gets talked about
- Damage your sperm's very structure and shape, so they are poorer in quality and less likely to be able to fertilize an egg
- Increase the risk of miscarriage if your partner does get pregnant. If a sperm cell is damaged but still manages to fertilize an egg, the result is more likely to be an embryo or fetus which 'isn't right' in some way. The mother's body is primed to recognize this, and end the pregnancy by miscarrying.

Fathers who smoke also have twice the risk of having babies with genetic defects. According to a German study of 8,000 births in 1983, these include a cleft palate (hare lip), heart defects and urinary tract problems. They are also more likely to develop childhood leukaemia and brain tumours.

Temperature check

Sperm hate heat. That is why their storage place is outside the body in the biological equivalent of a cool bag. The ideal temperature for sperm production is just 32°C (89.6°F), below normal body temperature at 37°C (98.4°F). If the temperature of the testes is even a degree too high, the stored sperm start dying off in their millions.

Excess heat can affect sperm so fast that men taking a nice hot bath for half an hour a day have been found to have lower sperm counts than normal – so beware the end-of-the-day hot soak. Steer clear too of luxuriating in a hot jacuzzi, sauna or steam bath.

Over-heated testicles are a work-related hazard too. Men in jobs involving exposure to heat, such as fire-fighting, welding, bakery or industrial laundry work, need to take regular breaks in cooler air, wear loose, cool clothing and have a cool shower after work. Long hours sitting at a desk or driving have a similar effect. Office workers and any-one whose job involves a lot of driving need to take similar precautions.

Varicoceles

Varicoceles are varicose veins within the scrotum itself. It is thought they may raise the temperature of the testes slightly, and so may affect sperm production. Studies have shown that about half of all the men surveyed with varicoceles had sperm abnormalities. These abnormalities disappeared for between a third and a half of them once the veins were removed.

However, urologists and fertility specialists disagree over whether testicular varicose veins are worth doing anything about, as many men with a varicocele or two are perfectly fertile and the condition is common. In one study of army recruits having their traditional physical check-up ('Cough, soldier!') 15% had these enlarged veins.

Infections, old and new

General infections of your urinary tract and prostate (prostastitis), even if they have all cleared up, may have done some damage in the past which could be affecting your fertility now. Some can stay around at a very low, subclinical level, not giving you any symptoms but detectable on medical tests. The same goes for sexually transmitted infections like chlamydia and NSU (non-specific urethritis). NSU is an infection or inflammation of the tube that brings urine from bladder to penis tip. It has been linked with poor sperm movement, more abnormal sperm and low sperm count. Any one of several bugs can cause the infection and if you are told you have NSU you need to find out which one. A GU clinic may be the best place for this.

If you are planning to start a family, it is a good idea to pay a visit to a GU clinic anyway before you begin, for a complete check-up, especially if you have ever had any such infections in the past, or if you notice any discharge or soreness at the end of your penis or when you urinate. In most clinics you don't need a referral, you can just turn up.

The pioneering preconceptual care organization Foresight recommends that men ask for a blanket precautionary check for *all* of the following bugs: gonorrhoea, group B streptococci, chlamydia, mycoplasma, ureaplasma, enterococcus, herpes, anaerobic bacteria, *Staphylococcus aureus*, *Haemophilus influenzae*, haemolytic streptococci, *Escherichia coli*, *Klebsiella*, *Gardnerella* and *Candida*.

It is a good idea to be checked for toxoplasmosis and cytomegalovirus too. Although these are not GU infections, they can play havoc with your fertility. The GU clinic may be prepared to pass some of your blood sample on to the appropriate department for testing.

You should also have your immunity to rubella (German measles) checked, because if you catch it and pass it to a pregnant female partner who is not immune either this can have serious consequences for the unborn child.

This sounds like a lot, but you might be surprised what can lurk down there unnoticed for years. Some of the above are 'minor' infections which do not show up much (sometimes not at all) in the way of symptoms, or they may be leftovers from previous infections you thought you'd cleared up long ago or never knew you had in the first place. Yet all can potentially affect your fertility.

SSS TIPS (SAVING SITTERS' SPERM)

- Get up and walk about regularly
- *Never* sit with your legs crossed
- Save tight jeans for occasional evenings
- Wear loose, cotton underwear

All the above are good tips for anyone trying to improve their sperm count, no matter where they work.

WHY 'SILENT' INFECTIONS MATTER
If your sperm is infected, even at a subclinical (mild, symptomless) level, it can make all the difference between being able to help create a successful pregnancy – and not. One survey found that in a group of 22 couples with fertility problems nine of the men had one or more infections in their semen.

Fertility foods – are you getting enough?

The standard medical advice is that you should get all the nutrients you need from a 'good balanced diet'. Unfortunately, most of us don't have one. In the UK the National Food Survey in 1995 found that the average person is seriously deficient in six out of ten common vitamins and minerals. This is not surprising. As life has become busier for most, the amount of convenience foods we eat has shot up. At the same time, the vitamin and mineral content of the fresh foods we buy has been dropping.

This decrease in nutritional value has been happening since the 1940s. According to joint research by the Royal Society of Chemistry and the Ministry of Agriculture, Fisheries and Food, between 1940 and 1990 vegetables in the UK lost 76% of their natural copper content, 24% of their magnesium and 27% of their iron quotient. From the vitamin point of view, it may be so long since an orange was picked that by the time you take it home from the supermarket it has lost most of the vitamin C you bought it for in the first place.

This is a problem because the food you eat affects every single cell and system in your entire body, providing the vital basic building blocks for your body's upkeep. The food and nourishment you take in is also needed for the production of healthy sperm, and for the development of your baby when you are pregnant.

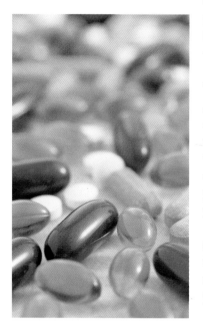

ABOVE Many minerals and vitamins that are important for fertility and pregnancy are quite fragile and easily destroyed by heat, cooking, light and storage – especially the B group (see page 51). Try to eat nutrient-rich fruit and veg raw and as fresh as possible, and consider taking good quality supplements.

Pro-fertility nutrients

For optimum health, everyone needs a wide range of nutrients – fats, proteins, sugars, trace elements and vitamins – in a delicate balance. Yet some nutrients are especially useful for fertility, both the mother's and the father's. Important ones for both sexes include vitamins A, B complex, magnesium, zinc, selenium, calcium, vitamin E and manganese.

ZINC

Zinc is needed for healthy sperm production, may help sperm penetrate the egg, and research suggests it can raise low testosterone levels by 150%. It's also important for the development of unborn babies. Shortage of zinc in pregnancy raises the risk of growth retardation, compromised mental development, malformations, more complications for the mother, longer labour and abnormal delivery. *Good sources*: seafood, wholegrains, dairy products and meat.

SELENIUM

This mineral is used to make antioxidants called selenoproteins which help protect the body from free radical cell damage – very important during the process of cell division. Deficiency in women has been linked with a higher miscarriage risk. For men, a lack of selenium is associated

> **SEX VITAMINS**
> Zinc can raise men's testosterone levels and B6 boosts women's fertility.

with sperm that cannot move properly, because the mineral is essential for making their strong whiplash tails. *Good sources*: fish (especially mackerel, herring and kippers), meat, wholemeal flour and anything made from it.

MANGANESE
Early studies on animals showed that this mineral is vital for ovulation and the maintenance of healthy testes. A lack of it leads to testicular degeneration, sterility, loss of libido and a higher risk of neonatal death. *Good sources*: tea, nuts, wholegrains and legumes.

ESSENTIAL FATTY ACIDS (EFAS)
Important for just about every system in the body, including the reproductive system. EFAs are used to make substances called prostaglandins, which have a hormone-like function. 'Good-quality' semen samples are rich in prostaglandins; poor-quality ones, whose sperm travel slowly and have a high level of deformity, are not. *Good sources*: there are two sorts of EFA: GLA (gamma linoleic acid), which comes from evening primrose oil, starflower oil, blackcurrant seed oil and borage oil; and omega 3, which comes from fish oil.

B VITAMINS
Some studies suggest that B6 may help boost women's fertility. One group of women whose periods had stopped due to hormonal imbalance were given B6 supplements for four months and for some of them their periods restarted. In another small study, 12 out of 14 women who had been trying to have a baby for up to seven years without success became pregnant at last after taking B6 for six months. Vitamin B12 has been shown to improve men's sperm count. *Good sources*: avocados, lentils, watermelon (B6); sardines, eggs, spirulina and seaweed (B12).

VITAMIN E
This is a strong antioxidant that fights free radical particles, high levels of which can damage sperm's precious DNA. The vitamin has had some success being used to help treat unexplained infertility in both men and women. If you do take it as a supplement, make sure you have the natural version called *d*-alpha-tocopherol, rather than the synthetic version, *dl*-alpha-tocopherol. The natural vitamin is easier to absorb and works more efficiently. *Good sources*: wheatgerm and unrefined cereal grains.

VITAMIN C
Research shows that vitamin C is good for sperm. Another antioxidant, it protects the sperm cells and the precious genetic material they carry from free radical damage. Clinical trials that involved giving one group of men 1000 mg vitamin C and others dummy pills showed the vitamin reduced the number of abnormal sperm, improved their movement and increased sperm count overall by a third. Other research suggests that

FANTASTIC FOLIC ACID
Start taking supplements of this B-group vitamin before you try to become pregnant. Research confirms that folic acid can dramatically reduce the risk of spina bifida, which can cause serious disability. The general dose is 400 mcg daily (available from a chemist).

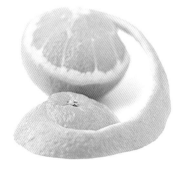
BELOW Fresh oranges have twice the recommended daily intake of vitamin C. If you suspect the freshness of the ones in your supermarket try tinned guavas or half a green pepper instead as they contain the same amount.

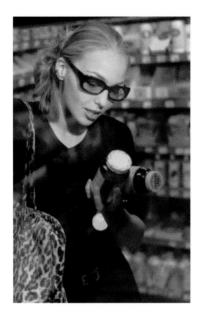

ABOVE Taking nutritional supplements may improve your health greatly and the range on offer at health food shops has never been better. But it pays to check what you personally may need or be short of, rather than buying a general pre-pregnancy or health-boosting formula which may cost you money and be of little use. Health professionals who can check accurately for you, using blood, sweat or muscle testing, include naturopaths, clinical ecologists, state registered dieticians or nutritionists.

daily supplements of 500 mg vitamin C stop sperm clumping together and free them up for the conception race. *Good sources*: tinned guavas, fresh oranges, green peppers, potatoes and green vegetables.

IRON

Supplements of this should only be given if you have had a blood test which shows you are definitely short of it. Iron deficiency, which can be caused by the blood loss of heavy periods, is always supposed to be checked as a matter of course in infertility treatment, because supplements have been known to help women who are having trouble conceiving. *Good sources*: include meat, poultry, leafy green vegetables and dried fruits.

Customize your pills

Before you hit the health-food shop to buy several bottles of the above-mentioned supplements, it is worth going to see a trained nutritionist or dietician, preferably one with a special interest in preconceptual care. Both partners need to go, as it will take both a good-quality sperm and a healthy ripe egg working together to create your baby.

Remember that, as far as vitamins and minerals are concerned, more isn't always better. If you take supplements of a nutrient you don't need, it will not necessarily have zero effect on you. For instance, too much of one could block the absorption pathways for another, creating yet another shortage. Very high doses of some of the fat-soluble vitamins can be toxic. On the other hand, too little of something you do need because you are short of it, or taking it in the wrong form, may have no effect at all. Furthermore, some nutrients are co-dependent ('friends'). For example, folic acid, which helps prevent spina bifida, and vitamin B12, used to make genetic material, work in partnership and you have to have both.

This is why professional advice is money well spent, if you can afford it. Taking account of both your health histories, the consultant will assess your needs and advise you on exactly what you and your partner would benefit from taking, and in precisely what doses.

WHERE TO GET ADVICE?

In Britain, state-registered dieticians who have a right to work within the National Health Service have a good three year's training; independent nutritionists have two to three years; a naturopath has an excellent grounding in nutrition and a clinical nutritionist is a medical doctor who has additional detailed specialist training in nutrition. Specialist nutritionists working for organizations including Foresight and the Women's Nutritional Advisory Service will be especially helpful.

Detoxing Your Food

If you are detoxing yourself and your lifestyle as part of a preconceptual care programme, you need to take a look at what you are eating and drinking. The trouble is that food just isn't what it used to be. It may look good on the supermarket shelf – shiny, blemish-free and colourful – but, unfortunately, much of it is no longer as wholesome as it appears.

To keep them pest-free, most fruits and vegetables today have been repeatedly sprayed with pesticide chemicals. To make breads last longer in your bread-bin, most contain preservatives. To grow meat faster, many beef cattle are fed artificial hormones. To avoid infections from their often cramped living conditions, chickens and pigs are fed antibiotics; in fact the use of penicillin on British farms is now eight times higher than it was 30 years ago. Inevitably, some, if not all, of these chemicals end up on our plates.

Xenoestrogens

Xenoestrogens – or synthetic oestrogens – are persistent environmental pollutants derived from pesticides and plastics. We eat them in our food, drink them in our water, and then store them up in our body fat. They disrupt the production and workings of sex hormones and can have a feminizing effect on the body, which is why the media has christened them 'gender-benders'.

Going organic – is it worth it?

This is a good question, since organic food can cost anything from an extra 100% to 300% or more than non-organic food, depending on whether you are buying a humble carrot from the local farmers' market or a succulent piece of prime free-range organic beef. Overall, the answer has to be 'yes', if you can afford it.

For one thing, organic food tastes better. But, perhaps more importantly for health, organic fruit and vegetables often contain higher levels of useful trace elements and are free from chemical pesticides, herbicides and artificial fertilizers. Organically reared animals are fed on organic food too, so they are also mostly chemical-free.

To cut the cost of going organic, try these supermarket alternatives:

- Join an organic food box scheme. A box of fruit and vegetables in season will be delivered to you weekly from local producers.
- Visit your local farmers' market. The produce will be loose and will not have travelled far to reach you.
- Buy locally produced meat. You may get a better deal on meat by going to an organic farm yourself or by ordering it via a butcher.

HOW TO PROTECT YOURSELF AGAINST XENOESTROGENS

- Eat only organic food.
- Wash all your fruit and vegetables thoroughly before use. Either use a commercially available fruit and vegetable cleaner (these are available as sprays and remove more pesticide residues than water alone) or add 2 teaspoons of vinegar to the bowl of washing water.
- Filter your water. Use a stainless steel filtration system fitted under the sink, not a plastic one. Alternatively, drink and cook with spring water, preferably bottled in glass not plastic.
- Reduce your intake of fatty animal products (meat and dairy). Xenoestrogens accumulate in fat.
- Never heat up food in plastic containers. Decant it into a glass or earthenware ovenproof dish.
- Don't wrap foods, especially fatty foods, in plastic. Buy fruit and vegetables loose and put them in paper bags or a wicker shopping basket. Ironically, most supermarkets sell organic produce pre-packed in plastic.

BEST ORGANIC BUYS
If you only have a little money to spend on organic food, the three most important things to buy organically are:

- *Grains* (e.g. rice, breads, breakfast cereals): As they are very small, grains have a large surface area to weight ratio and absorb more pesticides than other types of food for their weight.
- *Dairy products* (e.g. butter, milk, cheese, yogurts): Xenoestrogens are stored in ordinary fatty foods, yet organic dairy foods will contain few or none of these substances.
- *Root vegetables* (e.g. carrots and potatoes): These can act as major stores for pesticides.

If possible, buy organic apples and lettuces too – commercially produced ones are sprayed copiously and repeatedly with pest-controlling chemicals.

BE LABEL-WISE
If you are buying convenience foods, check the labels. The shorter the list of chemical additives, the better.

Although it costs much more you could perhaps eat less of it, using dairy or vegetarian foods more.

Your drinking water

The UK and USA's drinking water are among the cleanest and safest in the world. However, poisonous chemicals like lead from old piping can still sneak in, especially if your home is old and the area's water is soft. So can other substances, from nitrates to antibiotics and bacteria.

Even if the pipes are copper, they may be joined together by lead solder. Copper can leak into the water and high levels of copper are implicated in fertility problems. Water may also be contaminated by xenoestrogens.

WHAT TO DO?
Here are some suggestions to help prevent impurities in your water:
- Ask your local water board to run a check on your water supply for lead residues. Get any old pipes or joins replaced if necessary.
- Lead can leach into water just by standing in pipes overnight, so run the taps briefly first thing in the morning. Never use water from the hot tap for cooking, as lead dissolves more easily in hot water.
- Use bottled water (preferably stored in glass containers, not plastic) to drink, to cook with, and for hot drinks like tea and coffee.
- Get a stainless-steel water filter fitted to your water supply. Even though filters cannot remove every single impurity, they are a good start. Beware of the plastic jug type of filter – some experts suggest that the plastic can be a further source of xenoestrogens.

Detox food suggestions

- Think brown – go for unrefined complex carbohydrates (brown rice, wholemeal pasta, brown breads, rye breads), also millet, oats and rye. Avoid white bread, white pasta, biscuits and cakes.
- Drink pure water – six glasses a day. Add pure fruit juices if this gets boring.
- Reduce stimulants – avoid coffee and tea or limit yourself to one cup at your favourite time of day. Coffee has not specifically been shown to reduce fertility as such, but as little as two to four cups a day may delay conception, and a group of Swedish researchers found that four cups or more a day in early pregnancy doubled women's chances of miscarriage. Avoid caffeine-containing stimulating drinks too. Cut back on your chocolate intake – try carob bars as an alternative.
- Eat a leafy green vegetable a day. Cruciferous vegetables such as broccoli, kale, Brussels sprouts, cauliflower or cabbage can boost the liver's ability to detoxify harmful chemicals. The herb milk thistle is also said to be a useful detox agent (but not to be used during pregnancy).

The Fillings in Your Teeth

While on the subject of detoxing your body and your lifestyle, take a look at the fillings in your teeth. If they are a dark grey or silver colour – and the majority of fillings are – they contain mercury. Around 50% mercury to be exact; the rest is 35% silver, 13% tin, 2% copper and a trace of zinc mixed together into what is known as a dental amalgam. This lasts 7–10 years. When it starts to crumble, usual dental practice is to drill it without taking any particular precautions and then replace it with more of the same, unless you want to pay extra for a white cosmetic filling. Amalgam fillings have long been popular with dentists because the material is both cheap and easy to use.

Unfortunately, mercury is also extremely poisonous and, contrary to what most dentists would have us believe, it does not stay put in teeth.

MERCURY IN YOUR MOUTH
Mercury leaching into our bodies on a daily basis is not good news. It ranks second only to plutonium as the most toxic element in the world.

How does it get out?

Mercury vapour leaches out of our fillings and into the body all the time, when we eat, when we drink – especially if it's something hot like tea or coffee – and when we brush our teeth, because of the abrasion on the filling surfaces. Chewing gum is another good way to release it, especially as some people do this for fairly long periods at a time, to stave off boredom, aid concentration or help suppress appetite. Mercury is also used in root-canal treatments and may eventually leak out of these too, as the protective covering around them begins to break down.

Batteries in your mouth

Amalgam tooth fillings also do a good job of corroding themselves, according to a paper published by Professor James V. Masi, because they create a phenomenon known as electro-galvanism. This is a small electrical current in the mouth set up by two metals, one serving as a cathode and releasing positive charge and another serving as an anode. As it receives the charged ions, the metal acting as the anode gradually corrodes, releasing mercury vapour into your mouth.

Possible problems caused by mercury

Several hundred research papers and clinical reviews (we found around 70 in just one day's search, see References, page 136) have suggested that mercury stored in our bodies may cause a wide variety of symptoms and illnesses for both sexes. The list includes allergies, lethargy and constant tiredness, arthritis, ME (myalgic encephalomyelitis or post-viral fatigue syndrome), heart disease, mood disorders and mental problems including Alzheimer's disease, flu-like symptoms, tooth

OFFICE TIP
How can you release the maximum possible amount of mercury from your amalgam fillings? Chew gum and drink hot coffee while working at a VDU screen all day.

abscesses, chronic candida infection, eye problems, skin rashes, immune system problems, kidney disorders, period problems, reduced sperm count, ovulation disorders, miscarriage and premature birth.

The use of dental amalgams has been banned in both Sweden and Austria on health grounds. In Japan, though not prohibited by law, there is a high level of awareness about mercury poisoning so amalgam fillings are seldom used, and dental students are no longer even taught how to put them in. German dentists 'strongly advise' that the fillings are never used for children under six, for women of reproductive age or for anyone with a kidney problem. The influential British Dental Association does not, at the moment, officially accept that mercury amalgam fillings can be a health hazard. However, there are a handful of dentists in the UK, usually private, who are willing to work painstakingly to try to rid patients of these fillings safely.

How mercury affects fertility, pregnancy and unborn babies (see References, page 136)

FOR MEN

One study carried out in 1991 suggested that men who had been exposed to mercury vapour had 'significantly lower' rates of fertility. Mercury also impairs the making of the body's raw genetic material (DNA and RNA) and the process of cell division.

Published clinical research shows that mercury is stored in several places that are vital for men's sexuality and reproductive capability, including the testes, the pituitary gland, and the thyroid and adrenal glands.

FOR WOMEN

Several different types of reproductive and fertility-related disorders have been linked with mercury exposure. This may be partly because the poisonous metal accumulates in the pituitary gland, which is vital for stimulating the production of female sex and pregnancy hormones such as oestrogen and progesterone; and perhaps partly because, according to experiments carried out in 1983 on mice, it appears to build up in the ovaries them-selves, which store and ripen eggs.

Other research links mercury with painful and/or irregular periods, reduced fertility levels and premature birth. It is also implicated in miscarriage for workers who are exposed to it in their professions, such as den-tal assistants and women in

> **'HEAD-BANGING' SPERM**
> Animal studies suggest that mercury decreases fertility in men by affecting the way their sperm move. A higher proportion show 'head-banging' behaviour which makes it impossible for them to penetrate an egg even if they manage to reach it.

> **THE CONTRACEPTIVE KILLER**
> Mercury is such an effective 'sperm-zapper' that it was used in contraceptive gels and pastes sold in the UK right up until the early 1970s.

> **FILLINGS IN PREGNANCY**
> If a mother has amalgam fillings in her teeth, it continues to leak out while she is pregnant, crosses the placenta and ends up stored in her baby's body. It is thought to be especially damaging to the fetus's vulnerable developing nervous system.

certain types of factory work involving mercury compounds. When it was used to treat syphilis, 40-50 years ago, it was also found to induce abortions.

What to do

People differ in their sensitivity to all substances including toxic ones like mercury. And, among those who are sensitive to it, different individuals may react in different ways, suggest Quicksilver Associates of New York, depending on where any inherent weaknesses are within their own bodies.

One person might show mercury toxicity by having a weakened immune system and being highly susceptible to infections; another may have a finely balanced hormonal system and perhaps react by having ovulation problems. Yet another in their mid-thirties may show no visible signs just yet, but may turn out to be more susceptible to Alzheimer's disease or arthritis in their later years.

It can be a major undertaking to get your entire body mercury-free, and it will cost you money. If you are concerned about the possible effect of mercury poisoning from fillings on your fertility and future pregnancy:

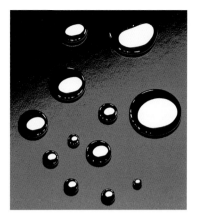

ABOVE Mercury is beautiful to look at but highly volatile and one of the most toxic substances on the planet.

- Try to read up as much about it as you can.
- Think carefully about your own medical and dental history. Might you or your partner have any of the symptoms of mercury toxicity? For instance, how many mercury fillings have you had? Are you having unexpected difficulty becoming pregnant? Is your partner's sperm count low, or does it contain a higher than usual number of damaged sperm, or sperm which swim oddly or not at all? You can get this checked via your doctor. Have you had problems with unexplained miscarriage in the past? Any chronic thrush (candida) infections that just won't quit, persistent allergies or feeling constantly tired?
- Have a small sample of stool or urine analysed to check out the levels of mercury in your body. You can send a faeces sample via a postal service to a reputable lab and you do not need a doctor's referral for this (PAMA, see Helplines, can advise).
- Have a full assessment of your test results and fillings carried out by a dentist who recognizes this as a problem and is properly trained and equipped to deal with it. These results, and discussion with a 'mercury-free' dentist or with a clinical nutritionist (a doctor who has specialist training in nutrition) will help you decide whether or not you need to take further action.

Getting rid of mercury

If you do come to the conclusion that you have a problem with mercury poisoning, the best approach is as follows:

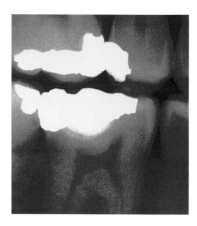

ABOVE What colour are your fillings – and can you remember how long ago they were put in?

ELIMINATION

Most elimination of mercury is done via the bowel, so this part of the programme tends to concentrate on maintaining good bowel movements (constipation is another side-effect of mercury poisoning). You may be advised to use fibre and gentle herbal laxatives, and to drink plenty of pure water.

DETOXIFICATION

You will need to consult a nutritionist or holistic physician for advice on how to do this, but it usually involves a nutritional programme to draw the mercury deposits out of your tissues. It may take several months.

There are several substances which help eliminate mercury from the body, and some work better for certain people than others. They include an amino acid called glutathione, vitamin B6, B complex, sulphur, seaweed, coriander, zinc, vitamin C, vitamin B1, selenium, activated charcoal and chelating agents.

SAFE REMOVAL OF AMALGAM FILLINGS

Amalgam fillings can either be replaced with gold ones or with white composite material. Some dentists prefer to remove the entire tooth because it is believed that dentine (the body of the natural tooth) also contains mercury and that this may still leak out even if the filling itself is removed. If you have root canals containing mercury, which may be leaking out, these can be evacuated and allowed to heal.

WARNING
Do not, under any circumstances, let a dentist who has no special knowledge of this area remove your amalgam fillings.

Proper precautions, including protection for your nose and mouth with well-fitting masks during the drilling, are essential during this procedure and many dentists are not aware of this. If these safety measures are not taken, you will inhale the mercury from your filling(s) while you are sitting in the treatment chair. This is because the heat generated by modern high-speed drills is enough to release the mercury in vapour form from the amalgam. Inhaling a large amount of toxic vapour like this may well mean you get worse instead of better. At the same time, you may also be swallowing small particles of the mercury amalgam filling.

The process of becoming mercury-free is a major undertaking, like pregnancy and parenthood itself. It can be expensive, depending on the number and type of replacements you have for old fillings or root canals. Filling removal and detoxification so your entire system is a mercury-free zone can also be a long process, and even after this has been completed it may be anything from a few days to a year or more before you feel better. However, it is also fair to say that the time it takes and the cost may pale into comparison next to several months' (or even years') worth of (possibly unsuccessful) fertility treatment.

Stress and Infertility: The Inside Story

Stress can be a powerful anti-reproductive agent at many different stages of the game. It can stop a couple conceiving in the first place, it can shorten a resulting pregnancy so a baby is born too soon, and it can affect the birth itself because, if a woman becomes distressed during labour or is afraid, the process tends to stop in its tracks.

Huge new international studies, like the EUROPOP 2000 study, have identified psychologically stressful work as a major cause of miscarriage and premature birth. There is also an effect on fertility. In several proven cases, previously infertile couples have suddenly conceived on their own when they neared the head of an adoption list or were at last given the go-ahead for fertility treatment. Many other studies have shown that extreme stress can stop ovulation dead, halt a woman's periods, and devastate both sperm count and quality (see References, page 136).

'Not getting pregnant when you are under stress or upset is an entirely natural – and perfectly rational – response to a situation which is making you feel unsafe or insecure. Something that a doctor would call "stress-induced hypo ovulation", not ovulating because of an excess of stress hormones in your system. Yet this isn't a disease. It is a normal response,' explains fertility counsellor Paul Entwhistle.

He continues, 'Females of most species need to feel safe in their nest to conceive. That means physically safe in your home, at work, emotionally and physically safe with your partner. When you are pregnant or caring for a young baby you are vulnerable so from an instinctive survival point of view you need to be assured first that you will be secure. If you aren't, your body may not risk you becoming pregnant in the first place.' Animals tend not to bear young when they are threatened or feeling unsafe, nor do they breed much in captivity. Why should we?'

> 'A number of studies show that if a woman becomes totally obsessed with wanting a baby she may even release eggs which are not mature enough to be fertilized.'
> *Preconceptual care practitioner, Dr Marilyn Glanville*

Twenty years ago most doctors sniffed contemptuously at the idea that stress and infertility were strongly linked. Even today, many still don't agree, despite the mounting evidence. And now those who do think it's true have found something new to argue about – the precise neuro-endocrinological mechanisms (i.e. how exactly does stress do it?).

The more enlightened fertility researchers like Dr Rosalind Bramwell of Liverpool University, and Dr Robert Edelman from the Roehampton Institute, UK, agree that stress is both a mental condition and a physical state, which has measurable, very real effects on a human's hormone-producing endocrine system – especially on its output of sex hormones.

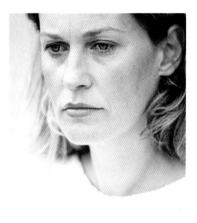

ABOVE Many people have had to become so used to managing pressured lives and long hours of work that this has come to feel normal. As a result they would not necessarily describe themselves as stressed, especially when they see their friends having to do the same.

EFFECTS OF STRESS
Prolonged stress can send women's Fallopian tubes into spasm, meaning that a fertilized egg cannot travel down to the womb.

These are the very hormones that drive fertility in men and women. Progressive fertility units, such as the Beth Israel Hospital in Boston, USA, have been including stress reduction in their programmes for 15 years.

The truth seems to be that if you have been feeling constantly stressed, and now find you cannot get pregnant, there are some cast-iron physical reasons for this. A psychological factor – supposedly all in the head – can cause several different biochemical problems, which are as solid as the chair you are sitting on. There is even a well-respected medical journal devoted to the subject, called the *Journal of Psychosomatic Obstetrics and Gynecology.* That's how real the connection between the mind and the reproductive system is.

Tackling sources of stress *together* (because even if it's only affecting one of you the problem it causes is a mutual one) can help you feel more in control, without it feeling it's somehow all your own fault that you are not conceiving together. See the sections on Emotional health on pages 42–3 and on Complementary therapies, beginning on page 78, for some suggestions of possible strategies and approaches.

How stress affects fertility

One of the reasons that stress affects fertility is that severe or prolonged periods of it can upset your pituitary gland. This little gland, about the size of a pea and nestled down underneath the hypothalamus just below your brain, does several different vital jobs within your body. As well as controlling growth, it's also the mission-control centre for your major stress hormones and sex hormones.

When it works well, it keeps everything steady, like an experienced conductor controlling a talented but slightly unruly orchestra. When it is thrown out of balance, however, the pituitary can produce all sorts of direct and indirect effects on your fertility and sexuality, causing symptoms from erratic periods to a low sperm count. It is well established that people with disorders of the pituitary (such as benign growths) experience infertility, but the gland does not need a major medical disorder to throw it into reproductive confusion.

BELOW There are concrete physical connections between stress hormones, the pituitary gland and the reproductive system.

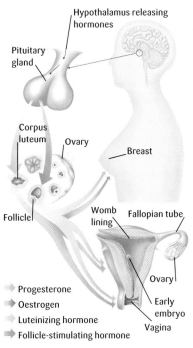

Hypothalamus releasing hormones

Pituitary gland

Corpus luteum

Ovary

Breast

Follicle

Womb lining

Fallopian tube

Ovary

Early embryo

Vagina

➤ Progesterone
➤ Oestrogen
➤ Luteinizing hormone
➤ Follicle-stimulating hormone

Sex and stress: what your pituitary gland can do

A woman's pituitary gland makes several powerful hormones:

- *Prolactin*: this stimulates milk production when breast-feeding. High levels can also stop ovulation and cause irregular periods.
- *FSH* (follicle-stimulating hormone) and *LH* (luteinizing hormone): these affect the ripening of eggs. Not enough FSH or LH means no ripe egg to be fertilized. No ripe eggs, no babies.
- *Oxytocin*: this hormone causes the contraction of the smooth muscle fibres and is responsible for making the womb contract powerfully during labour. Low levels may possibly compromise

fertility by affecting the muscle fibres in Fallopian tube walls, and in the walls of blood vessels supplying the womb lining.

- *Oestrogen and progesterone*: If oestrogen is not made in the right quantities, ovulation may happen erratically or not at all. If not enough progesterone is made in the second half of the menstrual cycle, the womb lining may not be thick enough or rich enough for a fertilized egg to implant, or the entire lining – egg and all – may be lost in a normal period.

Mutations

Not only can stress cause fertility problems, it can also prevent you from becoming, and staying, healthily pregnant. Some research suggests that stress causes infertility because it has a teratogenic effect on the gametes, i.e. it produces malformed eggs, or sperm, or both. Pregnancies created by a damaged sperm or egg usually result in miscarriages often so early you may not even realize you had conceived.

Other pieces of work variously suggest that stress affects testosterone levels, interferes with egg ripening and ovulation, or plays havoc with the delicate balance between the several female hormones needed for the reproductive cycle.

What happens to your libido?

For women, it's oestrogen and a small amount of testosterone that power sex drive. The pituitary has a direct effect on the first hormone and an indirect effect on the second. Higher than normal long-term levels of stress hormones such as cortisol and prolactin can have a knock-on effect on sex hormone production, and it's the same gland which makes them all. Low sex drive usually means you do not especially want sex. Not having much sex is a prime cause of infertility.

'Sex? Seems we are all getting less than we all thought. Fifty-five per cent of heterosexual men report they have intercourse once a week – or less – not the 'standard' 2 to 3 times a week.'
Men on Sex report, 1992

'The best way to get pregnant is to have plenty of unprotected sex. And I suspect not having much of it is a primary reason for fertility problems,' suggests Dr Bramwell. 'However it's not surprising that not being that interested any more is something that many couples don't like to admit to. Even to themselves. It's more acceptable to blame lack of pregnancy on a possible medical problem.'

No sex please – we're knackered

A new syndrome called TINS is seriously interfering with our sex lives. It stands for 'Two Incomes, No Sex' and it is now a common modern

THE POWER OF RELAXATION

Researchers at the University of Dublin were trying to help a group of women with unexplained (idiopathic) infertility in 1986. All the women had high prolactin levels, which can prevent ovulation. They were given relaxation training, their prolactin levels dropped back to normal – and their menstrual cycles gradually returned to normal too.

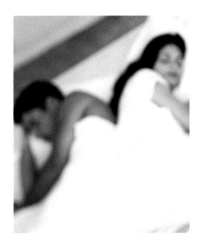

BELOW When you are tired and under pressure, the libido is usually the first thing to go. The bottom line is that you can survive without sex, but not without sleep.

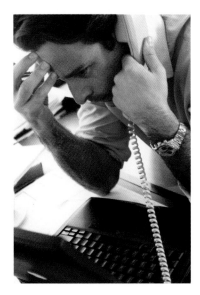

ABOVE If you are finding that it has become no longer possible to balance your work life and personal life, whether you are a bus driver or a bonds trader, it could be that you are no longer in the right job for you at this particular point in your life.

UNHAPPINESS CAN LOWER SPERM COUNT

One study of 157 men conducted by the University of California in 1997 showed that a very distressing experience, like the death of a close family member, can temporarily reduce a man's sperm count levels. Other research agrees that it lowers sperm count, and adds that it makes the sperm that are left move badly and can even cause sperm cell deformities. Undergoing infertility treatment itself can be such a roller-coaster that it may have a similar effect.

psycho-sexual phenomenon as love becomes the latest casualty of a non-stop culture. According to new research by a British organization called the Chartered Institute of Personal Development, over half of the people they interviewed said their sex lives were suffering because either or both partners were working such long hours they were far too tired to feel like it at the end of the day.

'TINS love fatigue' affects six-figure-salaried bond traders and lorry drivers equally. But, according to a recent survey by the Work Life Balance Centre, nurses are the worst hit, with two-thirds of them saying work was ruining their sex life.

Long hours are always stressful, and British workers clock up the most working hours in Europe, nearly 44 hours a week (the Euro-average is 40). At the same time, mental health charity MIND reports a British depression epidemic, and new fertility problems are rising – could the three be connected? The situation has dramatically worsened in the UK over the last two decades. In 1984, there were 2.8 million people doing really long hours of over 48 hours per week; now there are more than 4 million.

Men's fertility under stress

Men also produce the hormone prolactin, especially when under stress, and this can inhibit testosterone output, resulting in lowered sex drive, premature ejaculation, difficulty achieving orgasm and erection difficulties. If a man is under continual stress, there will be a constantly high level of prolactin in his system and that may interfere with the hormones controlling sperm production too. His age may also be a factor in reduced testosterone output.

Mood and emotions are controlled by the limbic system of the brain, which has a hotline to the little hypothalamus gland down below the brain's base. The hypothalamus is the central relay station for a group of chemicals called gonadotrophin-releasing hormone. These affect the production of the two hormones that play a major role in making sperm – LH and FSH.

Sustained stress is also a well-recognized cause of clinical depression, and depression is another enemy of both sexuality and fertility. The latest figures for the UK (2000) show that around half of all men and up to two-thirds of all women will experience depression at some time in their lives, and at any one time it's affecting up to 15% of women and around 10% of men.

If you are depressed you may experience a wide range of symptoms, from loss of appetite to exhaustion and sleep problems. As far as sexuality goes, many people also lose their desire for sex, and some report feeling little or no sexual pleasure when they make love. Depressed men may experience erection or ejaculation problems, or difficulty having an orgasm. Unfortunately, one of the main treatments, antidepressants, inhibits sex drive even further and can produce other sexual problems.

At Work

Do you spend half your waking life in a work environment, along with the majority of people aged 18-45? If so, the conditions there and the job you do are just as important to your chances of conceiving and having a successful pregnancy as your sexual health, the food you eat and when you make love.

Yet, because most of us work as part of a system with someone else as the boss, we often think there is nothing we can do to make our working conditions more fertility-friendly. Luckily, this is not the case. There are many important and effective things you can do, whether you are male or female.

For advice about occupational health risks, contact your trade organization or health-and-safety officer if you have one, or an advisory organization such as the London Hazards Centre. If your employer is being unhelpful, talk to your union, if you have one, or a solicitor.

In 1997, the medical journal *The Lancet* published details on a wide range of jobs and the possible effect on fertility. There are also many hundreds of other pieces of research looking at single issues, such as the effect of one toxin or hazard, or one type of job. Here are some of their conclusions.

Chemicals and toxic substances

EFFECTS ON FERTILITY

Women whose work involves contact with formaldehyde may experience sterility, reduced fertility and period problems. Those at risk include hospital staff and workers in the plastics, paints, foams, resin, and furniture-manufacturing industries.

The chemical carbon disulphide used in several manufacturing processes, such as the production of plastics, has been linked with sexual dysfunction in both women and men. Many pesticides and herbicides, including DDT, lindane and paraquat, are also known reproductive toxins. Some can lower sperm counts, others induce impotence. People working in gardens, parks, plant nurseries and farms are at risk.

Exposure to anaesthetics for health workers such as nurses, vets and dentists to metals like mercury and lead (from traffic fumes and cheap paints) in vapour form, to solvents (dry cleaning and lab staff) and to glycol ethers used by the electronics manufacturing industry has been shown to reduce sperm count, damage sperm or affect men's sex drive.

RISK OF MISCARRIAGE

Several substances and work-related hazards have been linked with miscarriage, such as anaesthetic gases for veterinary and dental workers and mercury for dental staff. Lead and its compounds are also associated with pregnancy loss, sterility, stillbirth and period problems.

YOUR RIGHTS

You have the legal right to ask your employer for a written assessment of any possible hazards to your health. Having identified the risks, they are then legally bound to take reasonable measures to protect you from them. If you are planning to try for a baby, this includes the effects your work may have on your fertility, your risk of miscarriage and your chances of having a healthy baby. Many jobs can affect one of the above, and some may make a difference to all three.

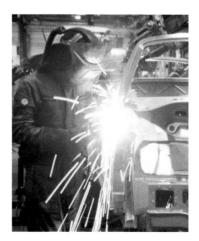

BELOW Many jobs for men involve exposure to heat, including welding, fire-fighting and working in a bakery. If you do one of these, take breaks in the open air, have a cool shower after work and wear loose cool clothing.

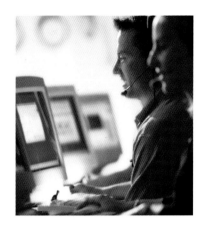

ABOVE Computers have revolutionized office jobs, but if you work with one each day it could be reducing your fertility. Try to take some – or all – of the practical precautions outlined below and opposite.

COMPUTER PROTECTION TIPS

- Take regular breaks away from the screen, at least 10 minutes in every hour.
- Try to avoid using the VDU for half your working day.
- Switch it *off* when not using it, rather than leaving it running on screensaver.
- Do not wear rubber-soled shoes or trainers when using the VDU as they increase static. If you have got them on, slip them off under your desk.
- Have the VDU earthed.
- If you are a freelancer and work, as many people now do, from home, put natural fibre (e.g. wool) carpets or wooden floors underneath your VDU.

continues on page 65

Besides workers who are involved in manufacturing processes, especially in the electronics industry, people at risk from lead toxicity at work include welders and anyone exposed to petrol fumes such as garage attendants, traffic police and traffic wardens.

There is some evidence that the pregnancies of partners of men exposed to anaesthetics at work are more likely to end in miscarriage.

THE UNBORN BABY'S HEALTH AND DEVELOPMENT

Women may be exposed to chemicals, such as solvents, if they work in a dry cleaners or in a laboratory. This may lead to a higher risk of fertility problems, miscarriage or having a baby with a birth defect or malformation. The commonly used thinner called methyl ethyl ketone can damage unborn babies in the womb. People who are painters, cleaners and lab workers are at particular risk from exposure to this.

Computer screens

Computers are not merely intelligent typewriters with glass TV screens that you can no longer run an office without. Their screens – or visual display units (VDUs) – also add potential hazard to the workplace by emitting X-rays, infra-red rays, ionizing radiation, static, microwaves, radio frequencies and pulsing fields of eight different types of electro-magnetic radiation.

The official line from the UK government's National Radiological Protection Board is that working with a VDU makes no difference to a woman's chances of conceiving and carrying a healthy baby to term. They point to evidence supplied by big studies, such as the one carried out in 1990 on 10,000 workers by the US Mount Sinai Medical Center with the research and campaigning group 9to5. This concluded that the 'apparent' link between VDU use and miscarriage was due to stress at work and 'recall bias' among the women. In other words, they felt the women who had problems in their pregnancies reported more potential risk factors when they thought back than women who didn't.

However, between 1978 and the early 1990s many other pieces of research came up with a link between working with a VDU and a wide range of reproductive problems. New studies on the subject are still coming out occasionally.

The reported problems include miscarriage in particular, but also period problems, infertility, a greater risk of babies born with heart defects and other congenital abnormalities; also of babies weighing too little. Many of these pieces of research were based on experiments with animal embryos, but some were large population studies looking at the experience of women working with VDUs in different countries.

The suggestion that VDUs might increase the risk of miscarriage first appeared in the 1970s with clusters being reported in Britain, America, Denmark and Sweden. In 1992 one particular study found that women exposed to VDUs with high magnetic fields had three times the risk of miscarriage. Another three-year study of 2,340 women by the National

Institute for Occupational Safety and Health in the USA found that female VDU workers were likely to have fewer successful pregnancies after a miscarriage, suggesting a possible effect on fertility or very early pregnancy loss.

In 1991, a Finnish review of a large number of experimental reports confirmed that the sort of magnetic fields associated with VDUs might well have a detrimental effect on the embryos of chicks, mice and rats. The effects included miscarriage and abnormalities. In several of the studies, the effect was worst when the embryos were exposed to these fields very early on in pregnancy. This is important because many women do not know they are pregnant for the first few weeks. Reports like these continue to appear. For instance, research published in 2001 by the L'Aquilia and La Sapienza Universities in Rome showed that ELF radiation stopped mouse egg follicles from ripening.

Clearly, even if the radiation emissions from VDUs are not 'causing' these reported reproductive problems directly, *something* untoward must be going on, unless, of course, all the clinical studies showing those higher rates of miscarriage and birth defects were (a) no more than a coincidence or (b) due to another factor connected with VDUs, but not the radiation, X-rays, static and so on that they give out. A number of other pieces of clinical research have, for instance, suggested that the potential stress of VDU work – sitting in the same position for long hours, repetitive work over which you have little control, often being under time pressure – may be the reason for higher than expected levels of fertility problems.

Some scientists suggest that men may be even more at risk than women from the effects of VDUs because their genitals containing their reproductive cells are external and therefore not so well protected as women's. Certainly the types of energy produced may be particularly harmful to fragile cells, such as immature sperm. Half-formed sperm are very vulnerable to external influences.

However, there is only a small amount of scattered evidence to suggest that working constantly with VDUs or in an environment where VDUs are in heavy use may have an effect on men's fertility. One Romanian study in 1985 looked at male technicians who had just been exposed to microwaves (one of the types of emissions from VDUs). Researchers found that not only was the men's sperm count lower but they also reported lower sex drive and problems with almost every aspect of lovemaking from erections to ejaculation, and even orgasm.

TACKLING THE HAZARDS OF VDUS

If there is a chance that VDUs may have even the smallest harmful but preventable effect on pregnancy and fertility, why not give them the benefit of the doubt and take some sensible, DIY precautions? There are now so many VDUs in use at work that if they really are a potential hazard, in any way whatsoever, they are certainly a very common one. And if something is common and it can, even very occasionally, cause major pregnancy and fertility problems, then it matters.

COMPUTER PROTECTION TIPS

continued from page 64

- Check regularly for any potentially hazardous radio frequencies. Hold a transistor radio tuned to VHF near the VDU. Wherever the interference is strongest, that is where any emissions are highest.

- Another way to check emissions is to leave a little vase of flowers next to your VDU and another several feet away, and see which wilts fastest. You can do the same with conkers (horse chestnuts) and check shrivel-time.

- According to the Institute de Recherches en Geobiologie at Chardonne in Switzerland, which has investigated the effects of radiation of a variety of plants, a cactus called *Cereus peruvianus* will help absorb some of the VDU's electromagnetic radiation.

- Sit as far away from the screen as you can, while still being able to sit comfortably and see it properly.

- Insist that your employers get good servicing engineers to come in and check the machines regularly.

- Place the VDU on cork-tile squares, rough side up.

- An ionizer on top of the desk may help.

- A big amethyst crystal on top of the desk has also been suggested. They are said to help absorb static.

Heat and temperature

As discussed earlier, excess heat kills sperm. This point is particularly relevant to men who spend a large part of the working day sitting at a desk or driving, as the sitting position keeps testicles warm. It's important to take frequent breaks, get up and walk about regularly, wear loose trousers and underpants rather than tight ones, and take a cool shower after work.

Attention: women at work

Certain types of punishing jobs are almost entirely the preserve of women. Work in the service industries, such as catering, retail work, teaching and health, often has a high level of contact with a demanding, often dissatisfied and sometimes even downright hostile, public. In the UK women make up nearly half the total workforce, but 86% of them work in these fields, compared with 59% of men. Teachers of big classes, nurses, shopworkers, waitresses, air stewardesses and supermarket checkout staff are all likely to face extra demands in the form of what's known as emotional labour. The air stewardess, for example, must remain calm, attractive and smiling, managing both her own emotions and those of her passengers no matter how she herself happens to be feeling at the time.

It is these high public contact and high stress jobs that place women more at risk of miscarriage, according to the big international EUROPOP 2000 study into pregnancy loss. They may also affect a woman's fertility levels because of their stress quotient.

Furthermore, women's workplace health problems are often compounded by going home to more of the same, especially if they have a family to care for.

There are many other women's work-related fertility hazards that are more concrete in nature because their levels are easy to measure. These include:

- *Vibration* - linked with irregular periods, which make it more difficult to become pregnant, miscarriages, birth defects and impaired hearing in the baby.
- *Stress* - linked with premature birth and also associated with problems actually getting pregnant (see Stress and infertility, page 59).
- *Shift work* - one 1993 study found that evening and night-shift workers were four times more likely to miscarry than day-shift workers. Night workers may also have more trouble conceiving if they work a mixture of night and day shifts since this can interfere with their menstrual cycle and ovulation.
- *Toxic substances* - see Chemicals and toxic substances, page 63.
- *Noise and long working hours* - have also been shown to cause problems in pregnancy.

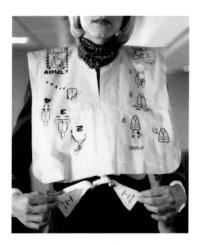

BELOW Being a flight attendant can be one of the most stressful jobs for women as it has such a high emotional labour quotient. This has been exacerbated by the aftermath of 11 September 2001, and the rise in air rage incidents and flight delays.

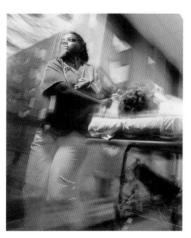

BOTTOM Nurses are in one of the most pressurized caring professions of all. The night shifts the job can involve may also disrupt their fertility and their libido.

Your Healthy Home

If you are about to move house, buy some new furniture, do some decorating, DIY, gardening, treat woodworm or eradicate fungi in your home, take a look at this section before you start.

We spend an estimated 90% of our time indoors, much of it inside the four walls of our own homes. Safe and sound, you'd think, from the pollution levels 'out there'. Unfortunately, we are not as safe as we'd like to think. In fact, according to a recent report by the normally reticent US Environmental Protection Agency (EPA): 'Indoor air pollution in residences, offices, schools and other buildings is ... one of the most serious potential environmental risks to health.' The EPA's study between 1979 and 1995 in New Jersey, North Carolina and South Dakota found that indoor air chemicals were five to ten times higher inside than out. In Britain, the Building Research Establishment conducted similar studies in 1996 and found that in semi-rural Avon air quality was an average of ten times worse indoors than outdoors.

They weren't just talking about the odd leaking gas pilot light or fumes from cheap new paint either, but about 'outgassing' from the myriad of new substances that have found their way into our homes in the last 40 years courtesy of the building, decorating, carpet and furniture industries.

The biggest group of culprits are called VOCs (volatile organic compounds) and they are made from petrochemicals. VOCs release polluting vapour at room temperatures. They are found in the ordinary building and furnishing materials used in most homes, including plywood, adhesives, paints, carpets, finishes, synthetic fabrics, household cleaning materials and wood panelling.

The two commonest VOCs are benzene and formaldehyde. Benzene is known to cause cancer in humans, and one major source is oil-based paints. Formaldehyde, which has been shown to cause period problems and infertility in women, is given off by glues, resins and preservatives; likely sources in homes are plywood and the adhesives used to bond pressed-wood building materials.

Having to worry about indoor chemical pollution on top of everything else may seem like the last straw, and to some it may smack of fanaticism. Yet the threat is real. Toxic vapours emitted by our houses and furniture which we cannot see or smell can and do affect us in many different ways, and exposure has been linked to a wide range of disorders from asthma to joint pain.

These emissions may be invisible but they can be measured all right, and often have been by organizations like the EPA. It has also been shown that some can affect a woman's fertility and ability to carry a healthy pregnancy to term. One particular American study in 1991 showed that a group of women with a history of unexplained infertility and recurrent miscarriage all had something in common – high levels of

DID YOU KNOW?
The Chemical Society registered its 10 millionth man-made chemical a couple of years ago. Health experts from allergy specialists to nutritionists and embryologists are becoming more and more concerned that we are showing signs of increasingly failing to cope with the 3,500 chemicals added to our food and 4,000 in our homes and workplaces. Some of these substances affect fertility, others may be a threat to the health of a newborn baby.

OUTGASSING
Ever sniffed the distinctive aroma of a brand new house? Then you know what outgassing smells like.

BELOW If you are decorating, check that you are using good-quality non-toxic paint, take regular fresh-air breaks and ventilate the room well both during and after.

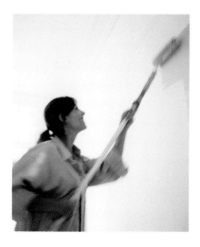

two chemicals that are commonly found in wood preservatives, leather upholstery and carpets.

What to do – simple, practical protection

The thought of our homes being potentially so polluted is not encouraging. Fortunately, there is a great deal that you can do to improve matters or even avoid the problem altogether.

TREATING WOODWORM

If anti-woodworm treatment is needed in your home, be wary of products containing the chemicals permethrin or lindane. Permethrin is commonly used to treat woodworm, and is also used in new carpets too. Unfortunately, it has also been linked with birth defects. Lindane is widely used as a wood preservative and anti-woodworm measure, and is also a known reproductive hazard. Research by the Faunhofer Institute of Toxicology and Aerosol Research in Germany suggests that house dust picks up permethrin and deposits it on food and kitchen surfaces, so you may end up both breathing it in and eating it.

Here are some suggestions regarding woodworm treatment:

- Try to get any woodworm treatments done before you move into a new house. Or move out when it is being done, and stay out for at least a few days afterwards.
- Ventilate the house ferociously before you take up residence once again.
- Move all foodstuffs not in tins or packets out of the house too. Store in boxes in a friend's house or in the boot of your car.
- Hire protective gloves and a mask from a DIY shop. Wear them to damp-dust and wash down all kitchen and bedroom surfaces, putting the cloths you use in a sealed bag in the dustbin as soon as you have finished. In fact if you have the energy, damp-dust *all* the surfaces.

DIY AND DECORATING

Try to get any essential DIY completed several months before you start trying to conceive. Some experts suggest four months, others say a year. This may sound alarmingly forward-thinking, but, if you are following even a basic preconceptual health programme and, say, giving up smoking cigarettes, recreational drugs and drinking booze for the recommended four to six months, then could you fit DIY projects naturally into the same time-frame or a little beforehand?

When it comes to decorating, be fussy about the selection and use of paints, cleaners and adhesives. Solvent-based paints and white spirit release gases that can stay around for weeks after you have finished. Many expectant parents choose to decorate their new baby's room shortly before the birth, not realizing that their newborn will be sleeping in a fog of potentially toxic chemicals.

Here are some suggestions regarding decorating:

- Use solvent-free paints and sealers that are water-based.
- Avoid cheap paint from extra-low budget sources: it may contain lead. Lead is poisonous, and exposure to it has been linked with sterility for men and women, miscarriage, stillbirth and brain damage in babies. Lead is banned in paint in many countries including the UK and USA, but cut-price paints from other countries may still contain some traces of it.
- Use a mask and gloves when stripping off any old paint – it may well contain lead. Watch for this in old painted furniture in particular, if, for example, you are restoring an old wooden cot or rocking chair for your baby's nursery.
- Decorate four to six months before you begin trying to conceive. Many couples feel it is tempting fate to decorate a room intended for a baby so soon. One way round this is to do the basics early on (e.g. put plain paint on the walls, lay carpets/flooring), leaving special personal touches such as friezes for the walls, lighting, pictures and curtains till a month or two before the baby is due.

FURNISHINGS AND FLOORINGS

Carpets are a major source of both benzene and formaldehyde, two of the most poisonous VOCs, especially when new. They can contain up to 120 different chemicals to retard fire, resist stains, kill fungi, stick on backing, stick the carpet to the floor base and discourage static.

Carpet outgassing is at its peak when carpets are new, but may in some cases persist for up to two or three years. In America the carpet industry responded to public concern about outgassing in 1992 by introducing a PR initiative called the Green Tag scheme, to show which carpets are supposedly low in VOCs. Unfortunately, animal experiments by the independent Anderson Laboratories, also in 1992, suggested that 'low VOC' carpets can still be pretty toxic.

Here are some suggestions regarding carpets:

- Limit the amount of carpeting that is used in your home. Consider more polished wooden floors, and cotton scatter rugs. Vinyl can also outgas.
- Avoid carpets treated with fungicides and stain-resistant chemicals.
- If you are buying carpet, choose some with latex-free backing. Do not let the carpet-layers glue it to the floor but ensure they use carpet gripper or nails instead.

ELECTRICAL APPLIANCES

Over the past ten years or so some health experts have become concerned about the possibility that electromagnetic fields (EMFs) may damage cells. EMFs are emitted by a wide range of electrical equipment, anything from your TV to that high-tension powerline outside the house. Studies have looked at associations with, among other things, leukaemia

TRY A BAKEOUT
If your home seems to be especially full of VOCs, consider doing a 'bakeout'. After your home has been built, renovated or redecorated, turn the heating up to about 38°C (100°F), open all the windows and run any ventilation system you have on full blast for two or three days. Leave the heating on overnight with windows shut, while you stay elsewhere. Ventilate vigorously before moving back in. Theoretically, this will encourage the materials in the house to release their gases quickly rather than over months, or even years. However, there is no systemic research on how effective this is.

BELOW Buying new furniture such as easy chairs or sofas? If possible, allow them to outgas outside your home for three days after they have been delivered.

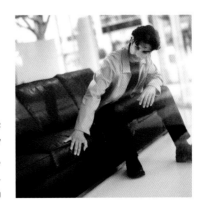

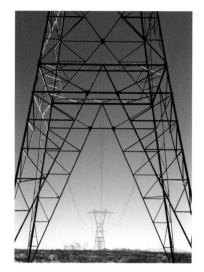

ABOVE Power lines and pylons are sources of electromagnetic (EM) radiation. EM radiation is the term for all the energy waves of the electro-magnetic spectrum. We are all exposed to radiation every day. Doses of all strengths have the potential to damage cells – especially vulnerable immature cells dividing in the body, like those of the ova, sperm and embryo.

CHEMICAL-FREE GARDENING

- Find out about alternative, non-chemical ways to discourage bugs and dis-eases. For instance, saucers containing beer are excellent slug traps and a line of garlic oil may deflect a column of marauding ants.
- Read instructions on the packet carefully, particularly if using chemicals on fruit or vegetables. Some pesticides should only be applied at certain stages of growth or so many weeks before harvest.
- Use non-chemical fertilizers and compost. The organic way is to feed the soil, not the plants themselves.

in children and cot death, but the evidence is still hotly debated. Although no links with fertility have been confirmed, it is worth noting that animal studies have shown that EMF frequencies between 15 and 60 Hz do affect cell protein-making and interrupt the synthesis of the genetic material called RNA.

As a simple practical precaution, it may be worth keeping EMFs to a minimum in the area we spend most time in when we are at home – the bedroom. Here are some suggestions regarding electrical appliances in the bedroom and other rooms in the house:

- Only use electric blankets to heat up your bed; switch off before you get in. Quite apart from their EMF-emitting properties, a bed that is too warm may make a man's testes too hot, thus damaging his sperm and reducing the amount he makes (see Temperature check, page 48).
- As an alternative, use a hot water bottle.
- Got an electric radio alarm clock right next to the bedside? Or an ordinary radio or CD player? Move it a few feet away.
- Site any low-voltage lighting transformers well away from your bedroom.
- Do not use a microwave oven unless you really need to. When it is on, stand as far away from it as possible (at least 1.5 m/4 ft is recommended) especially if you are already pregnant. Get the oven checked for leaks. *Always* turn the oven off before opening it up.
- Watch or use TVs, computers or games consoles from as far away as possible while still being able to see the screen comfortably.

Sources of EMFs occur outside the house too. It has been estimated that 100,000 homes in the UK alone may have high levels of electromagnetic radiation. Electrical supply cables may cause this, as might any pylons, electricity substations or telephone masts sited too nearby. You can check radiation levels with a hired EMF meter. If they are high and you feel this is worrying, consider moving house.

GARDENING

No gardener wants to see their roses buried under an avalanche of greenfly or to watch slugs waxing fat on their lettuces. Fortunately, these days there are plenty of alternatives to discouraging these garden pests with chemicals. Although not all pesticides and fertilizers are toxic to humans, and as with any poisonous substance it is the people who are exposed to high levels every day, perhaps through their work or because they live in highly polluted areas, who are most at risk, there is no doubt that some can be harmful. When the London Food Commission did a survey in 1988 of all pesticides then allowed in the UK, they found 35 that had potential to affect fertility and pregnancy.

Drugs and Medicines – What are you Taking?

Many drugs and medicines have an effect not only on a couple's chances of conception but also on an unborn baby right from the earliest few days and weeks in the womb. If you are taking any medication, even for a short period, and would like to become pregnant soon, always check with a doctor, preferably an obstetrician first. You may need to stop the drug or switch to another form of it, before trying to conceive.

Though this book is primarily about fertility and increasing the chances of healthy conception, we are including the effects on the developing baby as well because:

- Embryologists say that the first six to eight weeks of life are probably the most crucial for an unborn baby's development. During this time the embryo's developing system is at its most vulnerable to potential damage from toxins and drugs crossing from its mother's system.
- Many women are still unaware that they are pregnant at the eight-week stage.
- If a developing embryo or fetus is damaged by a drug or medicine crossing the placenta, it is more likely that the pregnancy will result in a miscarriage.

Medicines

All drugs have side-effects, but the fear that any particular one might harm an unborn baby has meant there has been relatively little testing of drugs on pregnant women compared with other areas of medicine.

Any drug or substance that can cause problems in an unborn baby is called a teratogen, or referred to as teratogenic, which means literally 'monster-forming' in Greek. The potential problems such a drug may cause include malformations, and restricted growth so that the baby is born smaller than it should be which can produce health difficulties of its own such as breathing problems. Certain drugs can also increase the risk of childhood cancers, miscarriage or even stillbirth.

Even some drugs that are known to be teratogenic often cause a pregnant woman and her unborn baby no problems at all. Different drugs affect different people in slightly different ways. This may be partly to do with how efficiently their liver can make enzymes to break the drugs down, and how much body fat they have for storing the drugs and their by-products. The mother's nutritional state is also important because if she is poorly nourished she will tend to clear drugs out of her system more slowly.

DRUGS IN PREGNANCY – THE FACTS

- On average, a third of women in the UK take medication which a doctor has prescribed for them at least once during their pregnancies.
- Most pregnant women try very hard to avoid taking any medication at all while they are pregnant. Nine out of ten will avoid taking even ordinary over-the-counter (non-prescription) drugs, no matter how unwell they feel.
- Just 6% take over-the-counter drugs in their first 12 weeks of pregnancy.
- Even drugs which are known teratogens do not always cause problems. The risk of any one drug causing a major congenital malformation is about 6–7%, or about three times the rate in the general population.

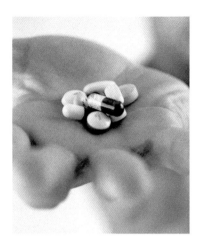

ABOVE Some drugs are best avoided early in pregnancy, but may be safer later on once the baby's major organs have developed and the risk of potential birth defects is lower.

According to a paper entitled 'Drugs to avoid in pregnancy' written in 2000 by a research and clinical team at the Department of Obstetrics at St Thomas' Hospital in London, if you are looking at the different causes for malformations '25% are due to genetic or chromosomal abnormalities, 10% to environmental causes including drugs – and 65% are unknown.'

Drugs to avoid

- *Anticonvulsants*: About 1 in 200 pregnant women needs to take medication for epilepsy. Unfortunately, some types of anti-convulsant drug increase the risk of the baby having neural tube defects like spina bifida, and heart problems.
- *Paracetamol* has been linked to mutations in animals and humans.
- *Antibiotics*, including tetracycline which is one of the most commonly used broad-spectrum antibiotics, can cause discoloration of the babies' teeth.
- *Sex hormones*: There is contradictory evidence about these. Danazol, for instance, a weak testosterone derivative, is often prescribed for period problems and endometriosis, but may masculinize female fetuses.
- *Anti-inflammatory drugs*: Non-steroidal anti-inflammatory drugs (NSAIDs) such as aspirin may increase the risk of bleeding in the baby after they are born. NSAIDs alone may affect the baby's kidneys and reduce the amount of amniotic fluid cushioning him or her in the womb.
- *Antifungal drugs*: Some used for fungal infections of the skin, hair and nails, should be avoided during pregnancy and discontinued at least one month before trying to conceive.
- *Synthetic vitamin A drugs (retinoids)*: Acitretin and isotretinoin, for severe psoriasis and antibiotic-resistant acne, are strongly associated with fetal abnormalities when taken orally. Acne treatment creams containing them have not been implicated, but women are advised to avoid them before and during pregnancy.
- *Thalidomide*: This infamous drug taught both the public and the medical profession a savage lesson about the potential for drugs to cause fetal abnormalities. It is now used for several conditions including a form of lupus and Kaposi's sarcoma.
- *Beta-blockers*: Used for high blood pressure and anxiety.
- *Ergotamine*: Used for migraine.
- *Nicotine replacement therapies* (nicotine patches or gums as stop-smoking aids).
- *Metronidazole*: Used to treat certain vaginal infections.
- *Tranquillizers*: Like benzodiazepines and antidepressants.

This list is not exhaustive. Please check with your obstetrician or doctor if you are taking medication and you either plan to become pregnant, or have already conceived.

'Benzo babies'

Benzodiazepines (BZDs) are commonly prescribed tranquillizers. Brand names include Ativan, Valium and Xanax, and they can be very difficult to give up. The campaigning medical newsletter *What Doctors Don't Tell You* suggests that there are one million adults in Britain currently addicted to BZD and a further million 'permanently disabled' by their attempts to come off it.

In the UK, it is estimated that there are 50,000 babies born every year to mothers who have taken benzodiazepines at some point during their pregnancy. If this is true (and it may be an inflated figure), that adds up to 1 in every 13 babies. However, to get it into perspective, 'taking BZDs in pregnancy' can mean anything from having been prescribed the drug as a one-off to having taken them the entire time.

In America, it is well documented that more than a third of all expectant mothers are given psycho-active drugs, including tranquillizers, at some point during their pregnancy to combat insomnia and anxiety. This is despite the fact that the UK drug reference books list BZDs as a drug to be given 'with special precautions only' in pregnancy, and the American Physicians Desk reference states they should not be used at all.

BZD taken by a pregnant woman can cross the placenta easily and will enter the unborn baby's system. Research studies suggest this could cause the baby to be born addicted to BZD in the same way as babies born to mothers who are hooked on drugs like heroin or crack are born with a physical addiction. These infants have been dubbed 'Benzo babies' by the popular media. Initial symptoms of BZD dependency in newborns include floppiness, agitation and inability to feed properly. However, a small number of experts suggest there could also be harmful longer-term effects.

Scattered research – which is by no means conclusive – suggests that potential additional problems for babies exposed to BZDs in the womb may include:

- A predisposition to developing addictions to drugs and alcohol as they grow up.
- More difficulty than usual in tolerating or dealing with stress, as their own natural calming mechanisms may have been permanently damaged. Research carried out in 1986 showed that BZD in the womb can destroy almost half of a baby's BZD receptors, the body's natural calming mechanism. One result of this is that the baby's neurotransmitters do not work properly and their levels of serotonin, the chemical which regulates mood, are always low.
- A tendency to develop attention deficit disorder (ADD). One study in 1993 suggests a specific link.
- Other problems for children reported in clinical journals include panic attacks and more anxiety and stress than is usual. This is thought to be because their self-calming mechanisms have been permanently harmed.

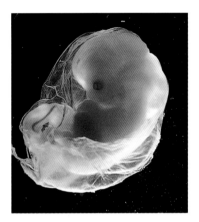

ABOVE This embryo is six weeks old. It has already formed a lifeline (two arteries and one vein) connecting it to the mother's circulation, bringing nourishment and oxygen in and sending waste products back out again. However, many different types of drugs can also come in via the same route, and may affect their developing system permanently.

BZD CAUTION
BZDs should not be taken for longer than four weeks. There are even warnings from the drug manufacturers in the leaflets inside the packets to this effect. Unaccountably, no such warnings are issued with BZD tablets which come in bottles.

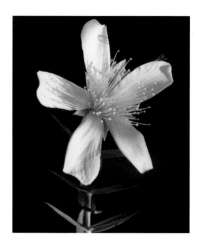

ABOVE Herbal medicines may be natural and work gently but they may still have side-effects, including unwanted effects on fertility. Like this one – the Hypericum flower. The extract of one of its biological variants *Hypericum perforatum* has been extensively researched and found to be a successful treatment for mild to moderate depression. If you are taking a herbal medicine and want to start a family, check with a herbalist or the manufacturer as to whether it can have a knock-on effect on your fertility potential.

The extent of the alleged damage depends on how long a mother was taking BZD for during her pregnancy, at what dosage; whether she was taking them for a limited period and at which stage of her pregnancy that was. Particularly crucial times may be during the first ten weeks, when all the baby's major organs and physiological networks are forming. According to San Diego-based psychologist Dr David B. Chamberlain, immediate Past President for the International Association of Pre and Perinatal Psychology & Health, the other important period could be during the second trimester, when the parts of the brain relating to emotional adjustment are forming.

If you need to take BZDs or any other addictive drugs at the moment and you would like to stop before you become pregnant; or if you are already pregnant, are taking the drugs and wish to come off them, talk to your doctor, obstetrician, health visitor or midwife as soon as you possibly can.

Herbal medicines

Natural medicines tend to work gently and have far fewer side-effects than manufactured drug treatments, but just because something's natural does not mean it is totally harmless – you get prussic acid from cherry stones. Herbs can be strong substances with a few side-effects of their own for a woman who is pregnant or a couple trying for a baby.

For instance, according to research by the Lorna Linda Hospital in California, the increasingly popular use of the herb St John's wort (*Hypericum perforatum*) for treating mild to moderate depression may also affect men's fertility. Their work suggests that the herb may affect the sperm's ability to penetrate an egg, and may even increase the risk of genetic mutations.

If you are taking a natural medicine, whether a herb or nutritional supplement, always check with a qualified herbalist or nutritionist whether it is safe to take it preconceptually or in the early days of pregnancy. It may be that you will need to stop for some weeks or even months before you try for a baby.

Street drugs

Many recreational drugs can also produce side-effects that can affect fertility and pregnancy.

CANNABIS

Cannabis increases the risk of complications during pregnancy, including placental abruption (where the placenta begins to peel away from the womb wall causing bleeding), premature birth, low birthweight babies and neonatal tremor (shakes in the baby).

Cannabis is thought to damage sperm production and to stop them swimming properly. As it reduces testosterone levels, it can also reduce sex drive, and has been associated with problems getting an erection.

OPIATES (MORPHINE, HEROIN, METHADONE)

Opiate abuse is known to treble the risk of miscarriage and stillbirth. It also quadruples the risk of premature birth. The baby may not grow well, and there is increased risk of sudden death after he or she is born.

Heroin damages sperm production, can cause a chronic drop in libido levels and can also inhibit ejaculation. Orgasm may be so delayed that a man has problems achieving a climax at all, which in itself would cause fertility problems. It is also associated with difficulties in achieving an erection.

COCAINE AND CRACK COCAINE

These can restrict blood supply to the womb, so the growing baby is deprived of oxygen and food. If a mother takes cocaine or crack, this has been shown to damage an embryo just three days after conception. Birth defects and low birthweight are associated risks. Exposure in the womb may cause psychiatric problems for the child as it grows up.

Long-term effects for men include an increase in the hormone prolactin. Resulting sexual problems include difficulty or inability to achieve or sustain an erection, and reduced libido. Cocaine use may also cause arousal difficulties and delayed ejaculation (some may have trouble ejaculating at all).

AMPHETAMINES

These can cause irregular periods, erratic ovulation and fertility problems. For the baby, the results can be heart defects, poor growth, stillbirth and premature births. Amphetamine use has also been linked with cot death.

Male libido drops with repeated use. Ironically, when one type of amphetamine, benzedrine, appeared in the 1982 edition of the *Handbook of Psychiatric Medicine* with a list of 39 things it was supposedly good for – one was impotence.

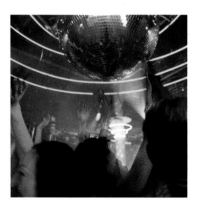

ABOVE The most popular drug in the urbanized West for the rave culture and long-term partying is still Ecstasy. No formal research has yet been carried out with regard to its effects on fertility. However, it has been shown to have other adverse health effects ranging from dehydration and morning-after depression to – in a few isolated cases – death.

STONED SPERM
American research at the University of Buffalo in 2000 found that very small amounts of cannabis make sperm more alert and increase the chances of them fertilizing the egg. Unfortunately, larger doses of its active ingredient, THC, make them 'sluggish, dopey and less likely to be able to penetrate the egg'.

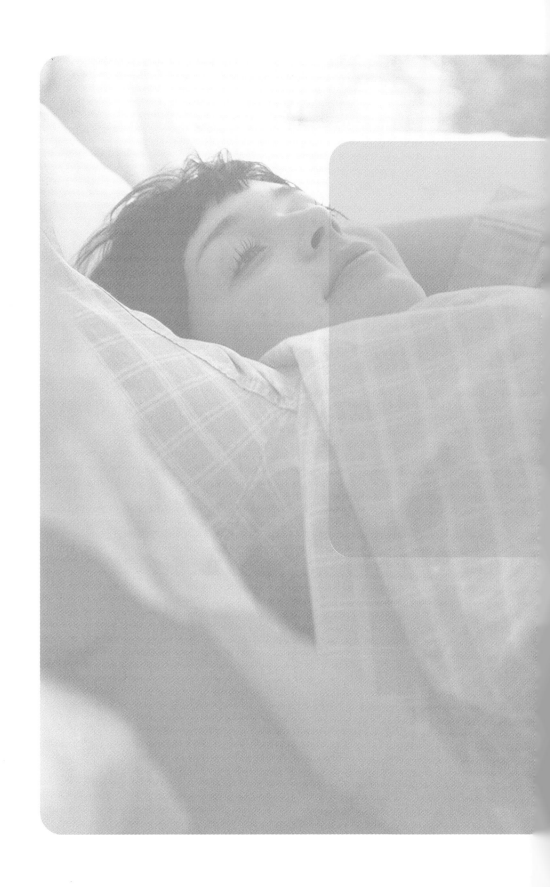

Complementary Therapies

There are many good reasons to use complementary therapies to enhance your fertility, not least because they have sometimes been effective in apparently 'hopeless' cases.

However, they are not the final port of call, a last desperate resort when you've tried every medical treatment in the book and none of it has worked.

If you are having problems becoming pregnant, complementary therapy, together with a sensible preconceptual case programme, is the very first thing to go for, not the last.

Why? Good professional complementary care – ranging from homeopathy to acupuncture – can maximize the chances of you conceiving naturally without costly medical help, and also optimizes the likelihood of any medical care you do still need to have actually working.

Complementary treatments are holistic – they look at you as a whole person in all your uniqueness and complexity. This means they take everything about you into consideration: your emotions, your job, your vulnerabilities, your unique strengths and the way you live your life, instead of focusing on a particular symptom in isolation, such as erratic ovulation. The therapies tend to work to find out the 'why?' that lies behind your physical symptoms, rather than merely suppressing the symptoms themselves. They also can provide excellent results at a fraction of the cost of ordinary (private) medical treatment.

Complementary therapies do not have all the answers. But neither does orthodox medicine. Both have a great deal of help to offer, but you'll get the best results if the two branches of medicine are working together for you, rather than when one is being used as a last ditch alternative to the other.

Homeopathy

What is it?

The word homeopathy comes from a Greek phrase meaning 'similar suffering', or that like will cure like. The treatment is based on three main principles:

- The *Law of Similars*. This states that the substance that produces the symptoms you have can also cure or alleviate those symptoms.
- The *Minimum Dose*. Homeopaths believe that to produce an effect or reaction you only need to give an extremely small amount of a remedy as a stimulus.
- The *Single Remedy*. Only one remedy is used at a time.

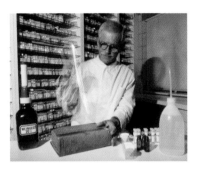

ABOVE During preparation of homeopathic medicines, the 'mother tincture' is diluted 1:99 with alcohol and shaken rapidly - a process called succussion, which is repeated many times.

For someone who is unwell, a homeopath prescribes minute doses of the substance or substances that could, in larger doses, produce similar symptoms. These doses may be diluted tens of thousands of times - so much so that no trace of the original substance can be found by any conventional methods of analysis. However, in homeopathy, less is more. The much-diluted substances are thought to leave behind slight echoes or vibrations of themselves, and the fainter these are the more powerful they are. This is in direct contrast to conventional medicine where the larger the dose of a medicine (usually a drug) is the more marked its effect will be.

Homeopathic remedies work by gently stimulating the body's own systems to encourage them to deal with any problems themselves without outside intervention. They are said to be helpful for almost all problems - both emotional and physical - unless any irreversible tissue changes have already taken place.

What does treatment involve?

A homeopath will spend anything from 45 minutes to an hour and a half taking a full medical and personal history, including not only your previous health and circumstances but also your personality and temperament, and finding out what sort of things make you feel better or worse. You are likely to be asked questions that may seem strange, such as 'Do you feel nervous in the dark?' 'Do you prefer mountains, or the sea?' as part of the practitioner's way of determining what is known as your 'constitutional type'. This has a major bearing on the type of remedy you will be given.

Homeopathic medicines come in the form of tiny white pills or powders. You put them under your tongue so they can dissolve. Do not eat or drink anything except water (especially not coffee or anything minty) for at least half an hour before or afterwards.

How long before I start to feel better?

Some remedies for acute emergency problems (for example shock, bleeding or allergic reaction) can work right away. For non-acute problems you may initially find the problem gets briefly worse (this is known as an aggravation), then you may start to feel better after a week or so.

There are a few basic general homeopathic remedies which are usually helpful, such as *Arnica 30c* for bruising and shock, and *Pulsatilla 30c* is often suggested for women whose periods are either totally absent or very irregular. However, the remedies work best if – like any complementary treatment – they are prescribed specifically and individually for the person concerned. For instance someone with irregular periods who had severe, needle-like period pains, often felt hot and began menstruating at the age of 11 would be given a totally different remedy from a woman whose irregular periods gave her dull aching pains, often felt chilly and began menstruating when she was 14.

Who says it works?

Several clinical trials have looked at the effects homeopathy can have on fertility and on disorders related to infertility, such as endometriosis. Two particular ones carried out in Germany suggested that homeopathic treatment may not only help infertile women achieve pregnancy but also prevent miscarriage. One study involved 119 women who were having fertility problems because of hormonal disorders. All were treated with homeopathy, 25 became pregnant and all but two pregnancies resulted in healthy babies. In fact, the usual miscarriage rate is one in seven confirmed pregnancies, so usually there would have been more than three miscarriages in a group of 25 women, suggesting that homeopathy cut the rate of pregnancy loss by one-third.

The other piece of research was done in 1993 and compared two groups of 21 women whose hormonal disorders were causing infertility. One group was given hormonal treatment and the other homeopathic treatment. In each group, six women became pregnant, but, while four of the hormone treatment group miscarried, none of the women who had been treated with homeopathy did so.

Some homeopathic remedies

The following remedies have all been suggested by Dr Andrew Lockie as examples of what a homeopath may prescribe for you, though he wishes to emphasize that for most problems, including fertility disorders, a personal consultation with your homeopath and a constitutional remedy are vital. Dr Lockie is a highly experienced homeopathic doctor who has specialist training in obstetrics, gynaecology and family planning. He is also a best-selling author. The following suggestions come from his book *The Family Guide to Homeopathy* (published by Hamish Hamilton).

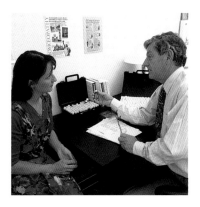

ABOVE A homeopath has more than 2,000 different remedies. He or she will take a very thorough medical, personal and emotional history from each new patient in order to choose one that not only treats the symptoms but also suits the patient's personality and characteristics.

MERCURY POISONING: A COMMON FACTOR IN INFERTILITY

Mild mercury poisoning due to leaks from 'silver' dental fillings is surprisingly common. It is also associated with a wide variety of fertility problems from abnormal sperm or low sperm count to recurrent miscarriage (see The fillings in your teeth, page 55). Symptoms which suggest mercury poisoning to a homeopath include feeling very sweaty, finding you have a lot of saliva in your mouth, and waking with small saliva patches on your pillow in the morning. The suggested remedy is *Merc. Sol.* once a week for four weeks.

NOT HAVING PERIODS (AMENORRHOEA)

The following may be of benefit if taken every 12 hours for up to 14 days. If your periods have not returned within a couple of months, see a professional homeopath. If you feel weary, weak, need to sit down all the time, your face is usually pale and you have occasional hot flushes try *Ferrum 30c*. If you find even minor emotional upsets disrupt your periods, you feel faint/shivery/weepy/sad, you have pain in your lower abdomen and a dry vagina, *Lycopodium 30c* may help. If you feel tired, giddy, chilly, your legs seem very heavy, your breasts are swollen and painful, and you yourself feel edgy and jumpy, try *Calcarea 30c*.

ERRATIC PERIODS (SUGGESTING ERRATIC OVULATION)

If it has been confirmed that the problem is pituitary-related, try *Agnus 6c* three times daily for three weeks out of four, stopping the week your period arrives. Note: the egg-ripening/releasing hormones produced by the pituitary may be disturbed by a number of things, including stress and even, occasionally, benign pituitary tumours.

HEAVY PERIODS

These are often caused by conditions which compromise women's fertility. Heavy periods featuring greater than usual blood loss, bad period pain, clots and dark blood at the beginning and end of the period may suggest either endometriosis or fibroids, so the following may be relevant. The remedies can be taken every eight hours for up to ten days, beginning just before the period is due.

If you lose a good deal of blood when you have your period, have abdominal cramps, feel nauseous especially for the first day or two, and if your pain and bleeding is worse at night, try *Borax 30c*. If the following sounds familiar – intermittent bleeding, losing dark clots of blood, feeling faint or giddy, bad abdominal cramps and your face looks very pale when you are menstruating, try *China 30c*. If your blood loss is bright red, you are also getting dragging pains in your womb, a throbbing headache and your face becomes flushed and hot when you have your period, try *Belladonna 30c*.

OVARIAN CYSTS AND POLYCYSTIC OVARIES

Again, a constitutional remedy would be best here, but the following may help too if taken four times a day for up to two weeks. If it's your right ovary that is causing the problem, your periods are painful, your lower abdomen feels tender and sore and you have stinging pains, try *Apis 6c*. If it's the left ovary and the pain is localized and worse in the morning but tends to wear off in the afternoons, try *Lachesis 6c*. For women who have lower abdominal pain 'which feels like a wedge has been driven through their ovary and womb', *Iodum 6c* may help.

FIBROIDS

If your doctor has confirmed that you have fibroids, rather than simply suspecting it because of your symptoms (see Heavy periods, above) the

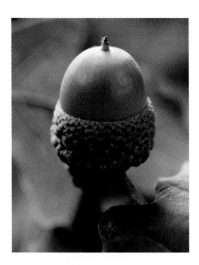

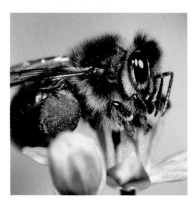

BELOW AND BOTTOM Homeopathic remedies contain minute amounts of a diverse range of natural substances. Sources range from plants such as oak tree acorns for the remedy *Quercus robur*, to insect venom, for example Apis made from bee stings can be used to soothe vicious mosquito bites.

recommended remedies are different. They should be taken four times daily for up to three weeks, and may include *Thlaspi 6c* if the bleeding is continuous or *Phosphorus 6c* if the blood you are losing is bright red. However, if your womb feels swollen, you are getting painful cramps when you have your period, you feel like you would like to 'bear down', and sometimes have some watery brownish discharge from your vagina, *Fraxinus 6c* is indicated. If you find your menstrual flow heavier than usual, bleed in between your periods too, and often feel icy cold, *Silicea 6c* may help.

INFERTILITY

For women, there are several specific remedies which may be taken every 12 hours for up to seven days while you are waiting for a full assessment from your doctor or specialist, and a proper constitutional treatment from a good homeopath. *Conium 30c* may be suggested if you find you are uninterested in sex, and your breasts feel tender and have some hard, swollen areas inside them. If you have had more than one miscarriage before 12 weeks, you may be advised to take *Sabina 30c*. If your periods are irregular, you feel chilly, weepy, and irritable; your womb feels as if it is about to 'drop down' or out of your vagina, and you feel a real aversion to sex, *Sepia 30c* may be useful.

If you have a dry vagina and your abdomen feels tender just over your right ovary, try *Lycopodium 30c*. If your specialist or doctor has found that you have a pituitary problem, the remedy *Agnus 6c* up to three times daily for three weeks out of four if your periods are regular, stopping the week of your period, may be suggested.

For men, again a proper, detailed medical examination and diagnosis are needed, and so is a good constitutional remedy. There are also however, certain specific homeopathic remedies which could be taken every 12 hours for up to seven days while waiting for the latter. They include *Sepia 30c* if you are conscious of a dragging feeling in your genitals and you have little or no desire for sex. If you feel cramp and coldness in your legs and find it difficult to maintain an erection for long, *Conium 30c* may be useful. If you feel you have become absent-minded, you lack energy and your erections are not firm, try *Agnus 30c*. However, if you feel more desire than you usually do to have sex but find that intercourse itself tends to be spoiled by anticipating 'failure', and you feel generally insecure, the remedy *Lycopodium 30c* may be indicated to help.

STRESS

Stress is hard to define. Not least because if it goes on for long enough it starts to feel normal, and one person's stressful office is another's stimulating, buzzing workplace. However, stress can be powerfully linked with fertility problems (see Stress and infertility, page 59). Homeopathic treatment for stress would be long term and constitutional, but for the short term, while you are waiting for an appointment with a good homeopath, see box right.

BELOW Many wild flowers, including the tiger lily, crocus, red foxglove and bluebell, are another rich source for homeopathic medicines.

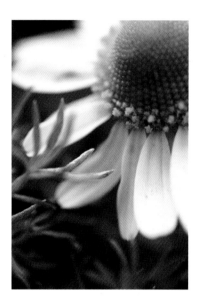

HOMEOPATHIC STRESS-BEATERS

- For stress due to an emotional upset or heavy personal disappointment - Ignatia 30c.
- For stress due to overwork - Picric ac. 30c.
- For stress because of having had some bad news, or due to grief or loss - Phosphoric ac. 30c.
- Stress due to burning the candle at both ends (also perhaps finding you have been smoking, drinking and eating too much too), and feeling irritable because of it - Nux 30c.

The above can be used four-hourly for up to 10 days.

Herbalism

What is it?

In its broadest sense, herbalism is the use of medicines made from plants. Herbs are probably the oldest form of treatment in existence, and they are used in almost every culture around the world. Fertility and the rituals surrounding it have always been very important in traditional societies where reproductive health was an integral part of general wellbeing, which may explain why there are so many good herbal remedies to enhance both fertility and sexual vitality.

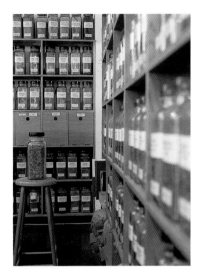

ABOVE Most herbal practitioners have a dispensary where they can make up prescriptions for their individual patients after a consultation. The remedies may contain just a single herb or a combination of two or three and are usually dispensed in tincture form.

Up until the eighteenth century herbs were the usual form of medicine used in the West, and even today one in seven of all conventional doctor's prescriptions are plant-based. Aspirin, for instance, was made from willow bark. However, herbalists feel it is safer to use the whole plant or at least a part of it rather than extracting and synthesizing only its active ingredients, then binding them together, as in conventional pharmacology (drug-making). Using the whole plant means that its active ingredients interact with its other constituents, which provide a buffering effect and help to counteract any side-effects.

As modern herbalists have become more scientific about their research, a new term has appeared to describe it: phytotherapy (plant therapy). In Europe, phytotherapists are usually medically trained doctors who feel herbs are both safe and effective. Organizations such as the European Scientific Cooperative on Phytotherapy in the Netherlands promotes the study of plants for clinical use.

What does treatment involve?

A herbalist will take a very detailed medical history on your first visit, which should last about an hour, and then give you the appropriate made-up herbal preparations to use at home. The prescription may be a single herb, or a careful mixture of several. Confusingly, the herbs may be called by several different names – their popular name, or 'country' name, their Latin name and, if they are from the Far East, their Chinese or Indian name too.

Herbal remedies come in various forms:

- An *infusion*, which is made from dried leaves of the herb(s) like a tea, and then drunk. Some can be quite bitter, so people often like to sweeten them with honey.
- A *tincture*, which is made by steeping the herbs in a mixture of water and alcohol.
- *Tablets* or *capsules*.
- A *poultice tube*, which is applied externally to the affected area.

Some remedies – especially for women

CHASTE TREE (*VITEX AGNUS-CASTUS*)

This pretty Mediterranean flowering plant is perhaps the queen of herbs for the female reproductive system. It is also known as chasteberry or monk's pepper. It can help regulate periods and balance out the oestrogen and progesterone levels and ratios. It does not contain hormones itself, but works by stimulating and balancing the output of the pituitary gland, which controls and stabilizes our reproductive hormones.

Chaste tree is also said to support the corpus luteum to make its vital hormones such as progesterone in the second half of the menstrual cycle. Helpful for menopausal problems and PMS, its uses in the fertility field include:

- Regulating irregular or painful periods
- Helping to control heavy bleeding and fibroid growth
- Re-establishing hormonal balance after taking the pill
- Keeping the hormone prolactin in check. Too much of this (often produced when we are under stress) can prevent ovulation.

It is also sometimes used before IVF treatment for women who might benefit from this form of assisted conception technique but whose follicle-stimulating hormone (FSH) levels are too high for it to be a success for her.

FALSE UNICORN ROOT (*CHAMAELIRIUM LUTEUM*, DEVIL'S BIT, HELONIAS ROOT)

Also known as blazing star, this herb comes from North America and contains hormone-like ingredients called saponins which partly account for its excellent reputation as a tonic for the uterus and the ovaries. It has an adaptogenic (balancing, normalizing) effect on the sex hormones and is often used to help disorders of the reproductive tract, period problems, endometriosis and PMS. Traditionally it is used for encouraging fertility in women, and alleviating potency problems for men.

DONG QUAI (*ANGELICA SINENSIS*, DANG GUI, CHINESE ANGELICA, TONG KUEI)

Also known as 'women's ginseng', this is probably the best Chinese herbal tonic there is for women, though it can also be used for men too. Valued highly in the East, it is used to treat the entire reproductive system and encourage the normal functioning of the sex organs. Dong quai should not be taken in early pregnancy (or if there is even a possibility that you may be pregnant). In the field of fertility treatment, it is used to:

- Regulate periods and ovulation
- Bring on delayed or suppressed periods
- Regulate the balance of hormones
- Stabilize the blood sugar levels.

BEING HERB-WISE

Herbs may be natural, but they are powerful substances which may cause harm if taken inappropriately, so they need to be treated with the same respect as orthodox drugs. You will get the best results if you go to see a qualified herbalist. If you are making up your own remedies bought at a health-food shop or by mail order, always talk to a qualified herbalist first. Some of the shops which sell dried herbs have knowledgeable sales staff running them; a few of them may even be trained herbalists.

AMAZING AYURVEDIC

Ayurvedic medicine is the traditional form of medicine practised in Sri Lanka and India. Like traditional Chinese medicine, it is a complete and complex system of health care. It involves the use of many different components, including herbs, exercise, detoxification, diet and techniques to improve both physical and emotional health, which work together to contribute to a way of life, and also as a treatment when someone is already ill. Its herbal remedies are called *Samana*.

Sophisticated and practical, Ayurvedic medicine's classic text, *Charaka samhita*, was written 2,000 years before the invention of the microscope. Yet it explains the body as being made up of tiny units (though

continues on page 84

AMAZING AYURVEDIC

continued from page 83

the text does not, as is often suggested, actually call them cells), lists 200 different microscopic organisms which may cause disease and accurately describes how disease spreads. Another important teaching text, *Susrutha samhita*, offers instruction on surgery, surgical equipment, stitching and the vital importance of hygiene after any operation. Detailed medical knowledge is interwoven with commonsense advice on how to live a healthy and fulfilling life.

There are two types of Ayurvedic practitioner in the West. *Ayurvedic physicians* are trained in India and often work within Asian communities. Indian training is generally of a high standard and is integrated with training in Western medicine over a six-year period, so the physicians are licensed to practise both types of medicine. An Ayurvedic physician should have the letter B after his or her name. *Ayurvedic practitioners*, on the other hand, are people who have initially trained in a Western discipline, perhaps medicine or a complementary therapy such as osteopathy, nutrition or herbalism, then went on to train in Ayurvedic medicine as well.

ASHWAGANDHA (*WITHANIA OMNIFERA*, WINTER CHERRY)

This is one of most important and respected herbs in Ayurvedic medicine. Ashwagandha is as valued as Chinese ginseng and less expensive – yet most members of the Western public have never even heard of it.

Ashwagandha seems to have a special affinity for both women's and men's reproductive systems. A famous rejuvenating herb, it is often used to strengthen an individual or some part of their body or tissues. It is highly recommended for treating weakness in children, the elderly and weakened pregnant women, as it is said to stabilize the embryo.

Ashwagandha is often given for stress, overwork, insomnia, physical and nervous exhaustion (which couples experiencing fertility problems may well have too).

LIFEROOT (*SENECIO AUREUS*)

Herbalists call this an 'emmanagogue', which means that it stimulates and promotes healthy periods and the normal flow of menstrual blood. Used as a tonic for the womb, it is prescribed to calm many types of menstrual problem, including delayed or suppressed (absent) periods.

Some remedies for men

SAW PALMETTO (*SERENOA SERRULATA*)

Also known as sabal, this plant from North America is prescribed as a nourishing tonic, especially for the reproductive system, and is a well-respected remedy for low libido, potency problems, testicular atrophy, inflammation of the reproductive tract and prostate enlargement. It can also be used as a reproductive tonic for women, increasing their milk flow, sexual energy and fertility.

YOHIMBINE

Made from the bark of an African tree, clinical trials have shown that this helps with potency problems, and male sexual vitality in general. Most of the research has been carried out on animals, but more is under way in America on humans. One particular trial in 1989, at St George's Hospital in London and The Hope Hospital in Manchester, found 'a significant improvement in the quality of erections'.

DAMIANA (*TURNERA APHRODISIACA*)

This herb is a valued a strengthener for the nervous system and also has an ancient reputation as an aphrodisiac, though whether the latter is deserved or not no one can seem to agree. It also has a tonic action on the hormonal system. The chemistry of the plant suggests that the alkaloids it contains may have a testosterone-like action. It's also a useful antidepressant, and is often prescribed for people where anxiety or depression may be linked with a sexual problem such as lack of desire, or erection difficulties. Damiana is also used to strengthen the male sexual system in general.

ASHWAGANDHA

See page 84. This herb is said to act as a general tonic to the entire hormonal system. Herbalists recommend it for low sperm count, 'sexual debility', and infertility and potency problems.

Stress-calming and relaxation

There is a powerful link between prolonged stress and fertility problems (see Stress and fertility, page 59) and so being able to bring down your stress levels and find regular ways to relax is an important part of any fertility treatment. Some progressive hospital clinics do now include anti-stress programmes for IVF patients.

All the complementary therapies mentioned in this book could help you deal with stress yourself to some extent. Reflexology, aromatherapy, Bach Flower Remedies, self-hypnosis, Autogenic Training, relaxation and visualization techniques, and herbalism can be especially effective. To promote relaxation and calm, a herbalist may suggest some of the following, either singly or in combination.

PASSIONFLOWER (*PASSIFLORA INCARNATA*)

The plant sounds as if it inflames sexual desire, but in fact it was named by the Spanish conquistadors and missionaries who found its exotic, purple flower reminded them of the thorn crown of Christ's passion. Both flower and vine are used to make a beautifully relaxing remedy. Passiflora is considered one of the very best tranquillizing herbs there is because it is non-addictive and allows you to wake feeling fresh rather than bleary-eyed next morning when it is taken to enhance sleep. It can be used to help support people who have serious disorders of the nervous system like Parkinson's and shingles – but also for agitation, stress, and any physical problem which is stress-related.

CHAMOMILE (*ANTHEMIS NOBILIS*) AND GERMAN CHAMOMILE (*MATRICARIA CHAMOMILLA*)

Also known as Roman chamomile, this plant's daisy-like flowers are used as a gentle and trusted relaxant for the nervous system. It is also anti-inflammatory and antispasmodic. The herb is a great digestion-calmer, because there is a powerful connection between the central nervous system and the gut (if you rolled all the nerve fibres threading through the gut into a ball they would form a mass the size of your brain). Chamomile's subtle sedative action makes it very popular for stress-related problems, anxiety, tension and insomnia.

WILD OAT (*AVENA SATIVA*)

This is used especially for nervous debility and exhaustion, or to support a beleaguered nervous system battling against stress, depression, anxiety, exhaustion or tension (see also Olive, in Bach flower remedies, page 89). It may also be suggested for people withdrawing from tranquillizers and antidepressants (see Benzo babies, page 73).

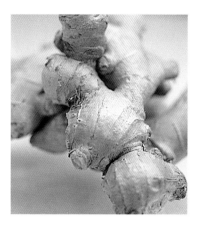

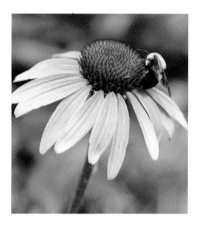

TOP Ginger is used to invigorate the reproductive system, relieve painful ovulation, inhibit excessive blood clotting (a cause of miscarriage, see page 119) and thin the blood.

ABOVE Echinacea is antibiotic, and it also stimulates the immune system making it especially useful for grumbling, subclinical GU infections – another common cause of sub-fertility for both sexes. The flower is a beautiful pink daisy-like bloom but it is the root which is used to make the medicine.

HOW LONG BEFORE I START TO FEEL BETTER?
You may notice an improvement after a week of taking a herbal remedy. Some long-term conditions may need several weeks or even months of treatment.

Bach Flower Remedies

What are they?

Few complementary therapies are as gentle and simple as the Bach (pronounced Batch) Flower Remedies collection. You may have seen these sets of 38 little brown bottles of flower tinctures on sale in health stores, and even in major high-street chemists. Based on the diluted essences of wild plants such as sweet chestnut, clematis and heather, they are used to help with emotional problems and states of mind, rather than physical disorders and illnesses.

GENTLE HEALING

The remedies' inventor was Dr Edward Bach, a bacteriologist and medical doctor working at the London Homeopathic Hospital, who gave up his lucrative Harley Street practice to develop them. He wrote that 'The action of the remedies is ... to flood our natures with the particular virtue we need, and wash out from us the fault that is causing the harm.'

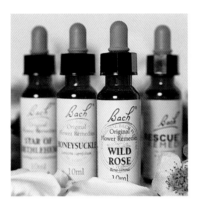

ABOVE Some of the most popular and best-loved of the Bach flower remedies: Star of Bethlehem for grief, shock and loss; Honeysuckle for those whose thoughts linger in the past or who cannot let go of something distressing that happened to them; Wild Rose helps those who are experiencing feelings of resignation, apathy or who cannot seem to become motivated after a setback.

Trying to conceive without results or going through a succession of the necessary invasive medical tests and medical treatments can be enormously stressful and tiring both physically and mentally. In uncertain circumstances like these, hope and positive thinking can easily switch places with powerful negative feelings like despondency, fear of failure, anxiety, mental exhaustion and depression. Bach Flower Remedies could be of great help here, as they gently tackle all these states of mind, and can subtly give you the support that you need. They do not interfere with any other type of treatment, whether complementary or clinical.

Therapists believe that the remedies do not work in a biochemical way as a herbal medicine made from a plant does. They are made not by steeping or boiling them to concentrate their essence as with herbal medicine, but by placing the flowers or plants in a glass bowl of clear spring-water in the sun for a few hours before removing them again. They are thought to leave an energy imprint behind, in much the same way as a homeopathic remedy does even after its original active ingredient has been diluted many hundreds of times over. The energized water is then bottled, and a little brandy added as a preservative.

Again, like homeopathic remedies, Bach Flower Remedies are thought to work by stimulating your own self-healing and self-balancing mechanisms. They work so subtly they have often been dismissed as worthless, yet those who use them report some profound – and lasting – changes for the better in their states of mind. The remedies are non-addictive, have no side-effects, are suitable for people of all ages and can be safely given even to pregnant women, babies and small animals. British independent (private) midwives use a composite Bach Flower called Rescue Remedy for women in labour and it is such a good calming treatment that it is also now a common sight in many office drawers, briefcases and home medicine cabinets.

Finding your type

Some Bach Flower Remedies are known as 'type remedies'. Your type remedy is essentially the one that is the most compatible with your particular sort of personality. Everyone's nature has a negative and a positive side. You take the remedy when the negative side of your character starts to overtake the positive.

The one practical problem with the type remedy is being able to analyse your own character without bias or undue modesty. You yourself might perhaps not be the best person to do this, especially if you are feeling stressed or low. To help find your personal remedy type, a therapist would ask you to think about the important events in your life and how you reacted to them. You could try asking yourself similar questions and just see what emerges. For instance, first take yourself back and try to remember how you were as a child:

- How did you feel when you first started school?
- How easy or hard was it for you to make new friends?

Now, bringing yourself up to the present day as an adult:

- How do you find you react to someone criticizing you?
- How do you cope with pain? With illness? With any crises that come your way? With setbacks?
- Think about your most important personal relationships at the moment, and how are you with these people?

These are all the sorts of questions that may help you find out your true nature. However, this is not a magazine personality quiz so you don't win any points for having one character type rather than another. No personality type is seen as being 'better' than any other – they just 'are'.

For instance, if you are a fairly extrovert person who speaks your mind, is impatient when held up and is a natural leader of others, remedies like impatiens or vervain could be most suited to you, but by a careful process of elimination you need to narrow it down to a single one. If necessary, ask a friend to help here. Try consulting a therapist who uses the remedies as they will have a good deal of experience in helping people pick the one which would suit them best. Some healers and homeopaths use a dowsing pendulum to do this.

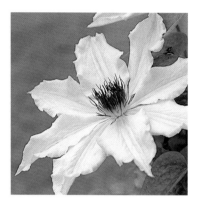

ABOVE The clematis flower – the remedy made from this is said to help those who are dreamy, absent-minded, living in the future, or who always need to have something to look forward to rather than being able to enjoy, and be fully aware of, living in the present.

What does the treatment involve?

The Bach remedies were developed to be straightforward to use, so that people could treat themselves. There are also therapists who specialize in the remedies' use. Many complementary health practitioners such as homeopaths, herbalists, spiritual healers, Reiki healers and aromatherapists are now also using them to complement their own treatments.

Each therapist will usually have his or her own individual way of working. However, an initial consultation can take anything from 15 to 60 minutes while they explain the system if you do not already know how it works, ask you questions about yourself and why you have come, and work out which remedy or remedies (as they can be used in combinations of two to six) might help you the most. You may need to

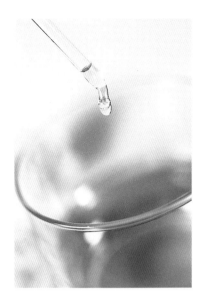

ABOVE One of the remedies being dropped into a glass of water, before being given to someone to drink.

HOW LONG BEFORE I START TO FEEL BETTER?
There can be an immediate improvement, but it may also take many weeks, depending on the nature of the problem. If you are self-prescribing, you take the remedy as and when needed.

see a therapist only once, or may find it helpful to do so several times over a period of months. The dosage rules for taking the remedies are fairly flexible. However, four drops in a glass of spring-water or two drops directly underneath your tongue three to four times a day are often suggested.

Some remedies

If you are experiencing difficulties conceiving, or are having actual fertility treatment at the moment, there is a great deal that the gentle Bach Flower Remedies can offer to support you.

AGRIMONY

This is for those who hide their feelings of considerable distress behind a strong or cheerful front. They claim everything is fine even when it isn't, which can be misinterpreted as not caring, or as taking important matters too lightly. Agrimony people may infuriate their partners by seeking the company of loud, cheery crowds of friends (pubs are ideal) to escape their worries. Their positive side is that they are genuine optimists, generous peacemakers and can truly laugh at their own worries because they see them clearly and in perspective. The agrimony remedy helps them to talk through their problems.

GENTIAN

This is for natural pessimists, discouraged easily even when they are doing well – but especially when they come across difficulties. They tend to suffer from depression. However, the positive side of a gentian person is terrific, believing there is no such thing as failure if someone is doing their best, and that no obstacle is too great, no task too big to be undertaken with conviction that it can be done. A gentian remedy encourages perseverance and provides the will to succeed.

LARCH

Larch is for those who lack confidence and cannot seem to help anticipating failure. If you are undergoing fertility treatment, the knowledge that the techniques have a relatively low success rate can be hard enough for any personality type to cope with, but may be especially stressful for larch people. Their positive side is that they are willing to plunge in there, take a chance with a hopeful and willing heart, and not be discouraged if it doesn't come off. The larch remedy encourages steady determination and faith in yourself, even after setbacks.

IMPATIENS

This is for people naturally in a hurry. Quick in thought and action, intelligent and intuitive, they tend to become impatient and irritable with those who are not as quick as they are, or when results don't arrive fast enough. For them, happy anticipation can soon turn to frustration and impatience. (When am I going to get pregnant? What's taking so long?')

Their anger flares up fast, yet dies away as quickly as it came. They may suffer from nervous tension, which often manifests itself as muscular pain, especially in the neck and shoulders. Impatiens can be useful for many types of pain and muscular tension caused by stress and anxiety, including pelvic spasm. Their positive side is great empathy, sympathy and gentleness for others, and tolerance or understanding for those less capable than themselves. The impatiens remedy encourages a calmer outlook, and more patience.

OLIVE

This is for those who are totally exhausted by long-term effort, or who have suffered for a long time under adverse conditions which have sapped their vitality. They now find they tire easily and quickly and seem to have no reserves of strength left to fall back on. Because they are so tired all the time, they find they no longer enjoy their work, or indeed anything that used to give them pleasure (possibly including sex). The positive side of olive people is that they know they can rely not on personal effort but on their sheer vitality to sustain and guide them. The olive remedy helps to replace lost energy.

PINE

Pine is for people who suffer feelings of undeserved guilt, who may find themselves worrying as they try to conceive: 'It must be my fault ...' or 'If only I hadn't done X, I might have been pregnant by now ...'. They cannot seem to help blaming themselves for mistakes others have made too, and they find themselves apologizing a good deal. The positive side is that a pine personality is willing to take responsibility, and to help bear the burdens of others if they can really help them. The pine remedy helps to stop those feelings of constant self-reproach.

WHITE CHESTNUT

This is for people tormented with persistent worries and unwanted thoughts preying on their minds. They cannot stop these going around and around their heads like a hamster on an exercise wheel. This could manifest itself as 'What else can I do?' or 'Who shall I turn to if it doesn't work out this time?' The positive side is someone with a calm, quiet mind who is at peace with the world and has learned to control their thoughts and imagination. The remedy helps restore peace of mind.

VERVAIN

This is for a person who is burning up with stress, tension, or sheer enthusiasm, someone who is living on their nerves, has very strong opinions, is highly strung and who will fret if they feel they cannot do all they want, or need to. They may be so anxious to become pregnant that they become very restless, cannot relax, and may experience a variety of aches and pains. The positive side is the wise, calm person who knows their own mind but is willing to listen to what others have to say. Vervain remedy encourages them to relax and slow down.

> **TRUE HEALING**
> There is no true healing unless there is a change in outlook, peace of mind, and inner happiness.
> *Dr Edward Bach*

BELOW Bach flower remedies do not act sharply or dramatically but work subtly. This change can come about within a few minutes (for example with Impatiens for anger) or it may materialize gradually, after several days of taking your remedy(ies).

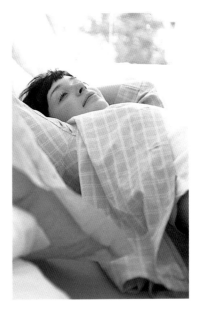

Traditional Chinese Therapies

What are they?

Acupressure, acupuncture and Chinese herbalism are all forms of traditional Chinese medicine. A practitioner may be trained in one or more of these disciplines.

TRADITIONAL CHINESE HERBALISM (TCH)

This is the use of Chinese herbs and plants to treat – and prevent – physical, mental and emotional ill-health. Often used together with acupuncture or acupressure, it forms the bulk of the Chinese medical treatment system, which has been used successfully for more than 2,000 years. According to the Chinese philosophy of yin and yang, acupuncture and acupressure are considered to be yang as they move from the outside inwards, and herbalism is felt to be yin because it works from the inside, radiating outwards.

Chinese herbs can be taken in combination – some medical recipes have as many as 12 herbal ingredients – and may be prepared as teas, pills, liquid tinctures, powders, pastes or ointments. In China, these medicinal herbs are very much part of everyday life. A Chinese person would tend to buy a herbal remedy as ready-to-use mixed dried herbs or in pill form over the counter from the herbalist, just as a Westerner might go to the chemist and buy a packet of paracetamol. Many of the patent Chinese herbal fertility medicines have wonderful names, like the Women's Precious Pills and White Phoenix Pills for women; or Five Seed Numerous Offspring pills and Lotus Stamen Combination (for exhaustion) for men.

ACUPRESSURE

Acupressure is the precise use of thumb or fingertip pressure on specific points on the body (the acu-points) which stimulate the flow of the body's natural energy (chi) along its designated pathways – the network of energy meridians. The Chinese believe that health and harmony depend on the unobstructed, continuous smooth flow of chi throughout the body. There are many basic acupressure points, some which are easy to locate. Practitioners often show their patients particular ones, or combinations, to press in order to help themselves when they are at home.

ACUPUNCTURE

Acupuncture involves placing very fine needles into the skin to stimulate the acu-points. These may sometimes be augmented by tiny electrodes (electro-acupressure) which some Western doctors like to use. Other important techniques include cupping, which involves placing bulbous upturned glass cups on the body's surface to create a vacuum over a particular point, and moxibustion, in which small

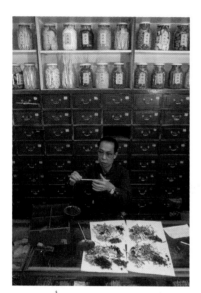

ABOVE This is how a traditional Chinese pharmacy often looks in both its country of origin and in the West. In China itself, the herbal remedies are also often dispensed alongside ordinary drugs in hospitals, or from street pharmacies.

SUITABLE FOR INFERTILITY
The World Health Organization has published a list of conditions that can benefit from traditional Chinese medicine, and infertility is one of them.

aromatic sticks or cones of a healing herb called *Artemisia vulgaris* (Chinese or common mugwort) are burned.

What does treatment involve?

A practitioner of traditional Chinese medicine (TCM) is likely to give you a very thorough examination based on four things: asking, looking, listening and feeling.

- *Asking* means taking a detailed medical history and finding out about everything that could possibly be relevant, from your lifestyle and sex life to diet and job.
- *Looking* involves checking the colour of your face, noting your eyes, complexion, expressions, the expression on your face, your apparent mental state and looking at your tongue (very important in Chinese diagnosis).
- *Listening* covers the quality of the voice, the sound of your breathing and the tone of your cough, plus the odour of both your breath and your body.
- *Feeling* refers to the checking of your pulses – something all TCM practitioners do.

In Chinese medicine, practitioners are trained to feel not one but six basic pulses which lie on the radial artery of each wrist. This makes 12 pulses altogether, each corresponding to a particular organ or function. There are 28 different possible pulse qualities. The old Chinese texts describe them as 'a pearl spinning in a dish', 'a tight lute string', fast, choppy or slippery. Your practitioner may also feel your abdomen for tender areas. This is called Japanese abdominal diagnosis, and is often used in Japan.

Who says it works?

There is a considerable body of medical literature, most of it written in Chinese, to suggest that acupuncture, acupressure and Chinese herbalism can be helpful for fertility problems in both men and women (see References, page 136).

One particular trial, published in 1992, was carried out on 45 women who were infertile, 27 of whom had very infrequent periods and 18 were not producing enough progesterone. The researchers matched them with 45 other similar women who had been trying to conceive for the same length of time and who had similar problems. The first group was treated with acupuncture via the ear (the points on the ear reflect the different areas of the body too, so treatment can be given by ear alone) and the second group was treated with hormones. Twenty-two women in the acupuncture group and 20 in the hormone medication group became pregnant, and only the hormone group had any unwelcome side-effects.

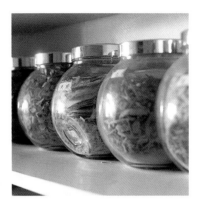

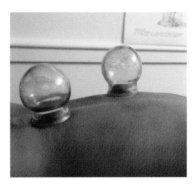

TOP Today, Chinese herbalists use more than 500 different dried herbs. Many are now available in pill form as the old-fashioned herbal teas can be notoriously bitter and time consuming to prepare.

ABOVE Cupping is another important part of traditional Chinese medicine and is sometimes used alongside herbalism. It involves small glass domes of varying sizes being placed over certain acupoints to draw the body's life force (qi or chi) to the area and thus encourage healing.

Another interesting study on infertile women at the Qian Fo Shan Hospital in Jinan, China, showed that 70% of women treated with acupuncture became pregnant within two years, 52% of those being treated with Chinese herbs alone conceived, and 46% of those being treated with conventional drugs. Yet another carried out in 1995 in China on eight couples with anti-sperm antibodies in their bloodstream used a recipe of Chinese herbs called Zibai Dihuang, taken in pill form. Pregnancy followed one to nine months after the treatment for all the couples. Another carried out in the same year, also in China, used the herbal combination Wuzi Dihuang liquor to treat male infertility. It was effective for all the mild to moderate cases of low sperm count, but not for those who had a severely low count, or a high proportion of abnormal sperm.

One particularly impressive sounding piece of published research, also published in 1995 in China, describes 202 cases of male infertility treated with the Shengjing combination herbal pill. After treatment, the quality and quantity of the men's sperm improved substantially, levels of the sperm-maturing and producing hormones were back to normal and anti-sperm antibodies reduced. One hundred and sixteen of the men successfully got their partners pregnant, and went on to have 108 healthy, well-developed babies.

In another study, the Chinese herbal composite remedy Nei-Yi helped women with painful endometriosis, which is a common cause of fertility problems.

Acupressure and how you can use it to help yourself

Sexual vitality is valued very highly in traditional Chinese medicine, not just as the driving force for the libido but more as an expression and regenerator of the precious life force which flows throughout the body (chi or qi). Sexual energy, if it is wisely used and maintained, can promote longevity and general good health. It is also believed that sexual energy charges and supplies all the major organs of the body, and that it also stimulates the workings of the mind and spirit. If your sexual energy is weak or low, it can lead to health problems.

Traditional Chinese medicine recognizes 12 main organs and divides them into yin/yang pairs which are described in terms of their function and the way they relate to each other. Each one refers to a complete set of functions, both physiological and psychological, rather than to a single structure based in one particular location like the heart or liver. These pairs are Liver–Gallbladder, Heart–Small Intestine, Spleen–Stomach, Lung–Large intestine and Kidney–Bladder, then finally Triple Heater and Pericardium.

The kidneys are thought to store the essence of life or chi. They are also believed to be the seat of vitality, endurance, intellect and creativity – and to house our instinct to mate, have babies and survive. They support the reproductive organs (ovaries, womb, testes and prostate),

---

HOW LONG BEFORE I START TO FEEL BETTER?

With acupuncture the improvement can begin after a single session, but, depending on what the problem is, your age and individual healing abilities, it does vary. However, you should begin to see noticeable improvement after three or four sessions. Acupressure may take between four and eight sessions to clear common problems, but chronic long-term conditions may require far longer treatment courses. With Chinese herbs you may feel an improvement after as little as a week, but for long-term chronic conditions it may take several weeks for any noticeable changes to begin.

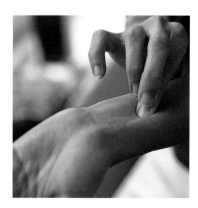

ABOVE Checking for one of the 12 pulses, which trained TCM practitioners can detect in the wrists.

their raw material (sperm and egg) and are the driving force fuelling desire, ovulation, ejaculation, fertilization and pregnancy. When kidney energy remains abundant, the person's sexual and reproductive life is both vigorous and long-lasting and their general health is good. This is why many of the traditional Chinese acupressure and acupuncture treatments for fertility problems involve strengthening the kidneys.

Useful acupressure points for helping promote fertility and sexual health and energy include the following.

CONCEPTION VESSEL 4 AND CONCEPTION VESSEL 6

For Conception vessel 4, measure four fingerwidths below your navel with one hand and find the point with your middle or index finger of the other hand. Apply pressure (gently if you have your period or your abdomen is swollen). This increases sexual vitality and potency for both men and women, and tones and strengthens the gynaecological organs.

For Conception vessel 6 measure just two fingerwidths below your navel. Apply downward pressure, gently rotating your fingertips. This helps increase general energy levels, and tones the gynaecological organs.

STOMACH 36

Find this point by measuring four fingerwidths below your knee on the *outer* edge of your shinbone (tibia). Place your fingers behind your leg for support and find the acupressure point with your thumb. As you apply pressure, angle it slightly downwards, towards the floor. This is a good overall tonic for increasing the body's general vitality, especially the gynaecological and digestive organs.

KIDNEY 3

Find this point on the inside of your ankle, in the small dip level with the tip of the anklebone. Place your fingers over the top for support and feel for the point with your thumb. It may feel a bit tender. Press, angling the pressure slightly downwards towards your heel. This strengthens the kidneys and the genitals for both men and women.

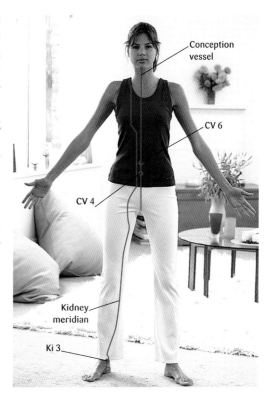

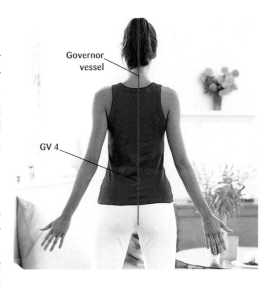

ABOVE A TCM practitioner would probably work on certain points along your Conception vessel, especially point No. 4 as shown, to increase sexual potency and to tone and strengthen the gynaecological organs. Another point for encouraging sexual health and optimum fertility lies on the Kidney meridian (energy line), and point No. 3 may be used to strengthen sexual vitality and to relieve anxiety.

Aromatherapy

What is it?

Aromatherapy is the use of the concentrated, aromatic essences extracted and distilled from plants of all types - flowers, spices, trees, herbs, fruit - to treat physical and mental disorders. There are about 150 essential oils, each with its own special scent and healing properties. Some, like tea tree oil, are antifungal, and some, like bergamot, are antiseptic. Others, such as lavender, help relieve pain and reduce inflammation. Many appear to affect the central nervous system and may have a calming, antidepressant or anti-anxiety effect. Hypotensive oils, such as marjoram, can help reduce raised blood pressure.

Instead of having one single property or quality, most of the oils have several. Eucalyptus, for instance, is antiseptic and decongestant, and is also a traditional vasodilator (it widens the capillaries and has a subsequent localized warming effect) so it is often used to treat aching muscles and sprains. Scientific research has identified many different chemical components in the oils that can exert specific effects on the mind and the body. Many more have yet to be identified as each oil has at least 100 different components. The substances we know of include:

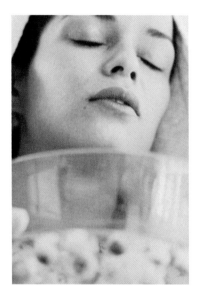

ABOVE AND BELOW If you need essential oils to work rapidly for you, try breathing them in as a steam inhalation. Their scent will stimulate the olfactory centres of your brain: the hippocampus and the thalamus. Both are linked to the hypothalamus, the part of your brain that controls mood – which is why aromatherapy can have such a powerful and rapid effect on the way you feel.

- *aldehydes*, which are calming
- *coumarins*, found in citrus oils, which are good for bruises
- *phenols*, which act as tonics (note that the body has difficulty metabolizing these and they may be toxic for those who are trying to become pregnant)
- *alcohols*, found in geranium, palmarosa and rosewood, which have a regulating, balancing effect and are helpful for re-establishing hormonal balance
- *esters*, which are very safe chemical constituents that have a calming effect on the nervous system.

The essential oils are used in various different ways:

- *Inhalation*: The oils (a) pass into the bloodstream via tiny capillaries near the nose's skin surface and (b) are converted into electrical impulses by the olfactory (smell) system, and finally are transmitted to the brain.
- *Through the skin*: Although skin is usually an efficient barrier, if essential oils are mixed with a carrier oil and used in massage, they can be detected in your blood and body fluids as little as 20 minutes later. This is because they can be absorbed via the hair follicles and sweat pores whose roots lie in the layer of the skin where your blood capillaries grow.

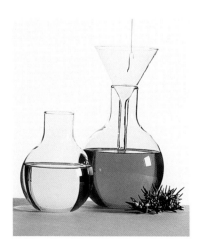

- *By mouth:* In France, only qualified medical personnel such as doctors and nurses are permitted to practise aromatherapy, and they may sometimes prescribe essential oils to be taken internally.

Who says it works?

Aromatherapy has been used as part of the treatment of both men's and women's fertility problems for many years, with numerous case studies and anecdotal reports testifying to the help it can offer. Unfortunately, we have been unable to find any published research studies of larger groups of people in this area, not even on the European *Essential Oil Research Consultancy* database in France which has collated more than 3,000 pieces of research into the oils, their properties and their biochemical constituents.

However, there has been a good deal of published research into aromatherapy used to correct other disorders, some of it so extensive that even the most orthodox scientists cannot argue with the results. One particular study was carried out by midwives in Cambridgeshire, UK over periods of eight years on 8,000 women who had their babies there. It showed that the mothers who used aromatherapy in labour needed 60% less conventional drug-based pain relief, and that they also had fewer episiotomies and tears.

In 1994 a strict randomized controlled trial was carried out on 100 patients who had recently had heart surgery. Half the patients massaged with oil containing essential essences and the other half used oil with no added essences. Patients in the first group were still reporting measurable health benefits five days later, but the other group reported none.

Using aromatherapy

Aromatherapy can be used in two different ways to help support couples who are trying for a baby naturally, or who have fertility problems for which they are undergoing treatment.

The first is to promote both mental and physical relaxation, which can make a very significant difference to your chances of becoming pregnant (see Stress and infertility, page 59). This may be especially helpful for couples who are trying assisted conception methods such as IVF and ICSI (intracytoplasm sperm injection), or who are undergoing a series of investigative and diagnostic tests to try to pinpoint any problems. The second way aromatherapy may be used is to help tackle specific health problems which are affecting your fertility, such as erratic periods or endometriosis.

Certain oils may also have a normalizing effect on hormonal balance in general. Rose, the queen of essential oils, is one which is often used for this and is said to work not by stimulating the female reproductive system but by regulating and cleansing it. There are others, such as fennel and anise-star, that contain chemicals with oestrogen-like properties, and these may also be useful for normalizing a woman's

CLINICAL AROMATHERAPY
Aromatherapy is increasingly used in hospitals and hospices. In the UK it is used in several different types of medical unit, including in the oncology (cancer), cardiac (heart medicine) and obstetric wards.

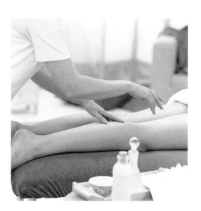

ABOVE A full body massage is the most deeply relaxing and sensual way to administer aromatherapy treatments.

ROSE FOR FERTILITY
Rose has long been a symbol of love, which was why petals used to be scattered at weddings to ensure a happy marriage. It is thought to be beneficial for men's fertility problems too (possibly by increasing sperm production) and aromatherapists say it may also be helpful for sexual difficulties.

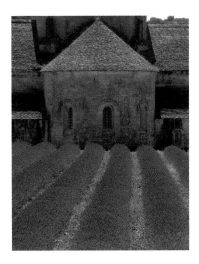

ABOVE One of the lavender fields of France. Lavender essential oil has a balancing and calming effect on both mind and body. It is also famous for soothing anxiety and helping promote restful sleep.

reproductive system. Note, however, that fennel is not considered safe to use during pregnancy and many aromatherapists avoid using it preconceptually too. Anise-star also needs to be used with caution as it can slow the circulation.

What does treatment involve?

An appointment with an aromatherapist will last from one to one and a half hours. Your therapist should take a full medical history and explore why you have come to see him or her. She or he will then choose the oils which they feel would suit you the best. The treatment itself usually takes the form of a full body massage with diluted essential oils lasting between 30 and 60 minutes.

Suggested oils to use at home

Couples who enjoy massaging each other could try relaxing, sensuous oils such as neroli, orange, bergamot and ylang ylang. Neroli is said have a calming effect on the nervous system, and also to be anti-spasmodic, so may also help to reduce any muscular tension in the pelvic area, which is often produced by stress. Spasm reduces vital blood supply to the area, and can even send the Fallopian tubes into seizure meaning that the egg cannot get down them. Orange has an uplifting, calming effect; Bergamot is antifungal or antiseptic and a favourite to use to help combat genito-urinary (GU) infections - subclinical GU infections are a fairly common cause of fertility problems for both sexes (see Bug-busting, page 40). Ylang ylang is indicated for sexual difficulties which are caused by anxiety and stress.

Especially good for women is a mixture of rose, lavender, neroli and mandarin - this is calming, delicate and uplifting and smells divine.

Essential oils can also be used in a vaporizer around the house. Try lavender and geranium to calm both mind and body. Put six drops in the burner's water and light a heating candle underneath every day. Place in the sitting room or bedroom at night if fertility issues, or indeed any other factors, are producing stress. For full therapeutic effect, vaporize these oils for three hours in the evening wherever you are sitting, before going to bed.

WHERE ELSE?
- *In a bath:* Add eight to ten drops of essential oil to your bath water (most people can't get a massage every night at home so this can be a good substitute).
- *Under a shower:* Add essential oils to a base shower gel, then use on a sponge or loofah for a wonderfully relaxing (or invigorating, depending on which oils you used) wash.
- As a *hot compress*, on a *tissue* (use 1-2 drops), as a *gargle*, a *steam inhalation* (3-4 drops in a large bowl of hot water), in *shampoo* or *moisturizing cream* (1-2 drops).

Reflexology

What is it?

This is no ordinary foot massage. Reflexology involves pressing, massaging and working very specific small areas of the hands and feet to restore balance within the body and help alleviate ill health.

Like auricular therapy (acupuncture which uses only points on the ear) reflexology is based on the belief that a small part of the body can be a microcosm of the whole, and can be used to bring about changes in those many other areas to which it is connected.

Reflexology also teaches that your body is divided into ten vertical zones, five on the left and five on the right. Each zone runs from your head right down to the reflex areas of your hands and feet, and from the front through to the back of the body. All body parts within each zone are thought to be linked by nerve pathways, and mirrored in the soles of your feet. The heels, for instance, relate to the left and right pelvic areas and sciatic nerve, the ankles to the reproductive organs.

No one is quite sure how reflexology works beyond the physical act of stimulating nerve endings in the feet. But one explanation is given in terms of the electrical energy which continuously flows though the nerve pathways of the body, which has been shown to exist by Western scientific research studies investigating acupuncture. Reflexologists believe that good health depends upon this energy being free to move, and that if its pathways become obstructed this can cause pain or dysfunction in the areas it should be supplying.

However, it is possible that reflexology works because the pressure of the therapists' fingers on specific sites on the sole of the foot or palm of the hand stimulates the nerve endings (there are 14,000 on a pair of foot soles alone). This is thought to send out small pulses of bio-electrical energy to clear any blockages, thus restoring a normal, uninterrupted energy flow and having a positive effect on the body's autonomic nervous systems.

Reflexology has had success in treating endometriosis, erratic peri-ods (suggesting erratic ovulation), non-ovulation and absent periods, polycystic ovarian syndrome, long-term stress conditions and anxiety states which can also disrupt the output and balance of both men's and women's sex hormones (see Stress and infertility, page 59).

What does treatment involve?

The therapist will take a careful medical and personal history first, then work on your bare feet as you lie back in a reclining chair or on a massage couch. Reflexologists use very particular ways of applying pressure or working the feet, such as finger or thumb pressure, small circular massage movements (rotating), 'finger walking' and flexing.

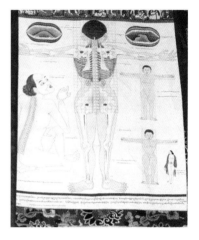

ABOVE Many cultures with highly respected and sophisticated traditional systems of medicine believe in the theory that invisible channels of energy (meridians) run through the human body. Above is part of an ancient Tibetan wall hanging showing their physicians' interpretation of the energy channel system. It's not dissimilar from the system that forms the basis of Chinese acupuncture and Western reflexology.

The session will begin and end with a relaxation treatment to relax the diaphragm, loosen the joints and free your ankles. The therapist will then work over the entire foot, and finally return to concentrate gently on any problem areas found.

If a certain area feels tender or painful to press, this suggests an imbalance or blockage in the corresponding body area or organ. The treatment is a gentle one and is usually calming and relaxing. However, working a problem area to encourage healing may be uncomfortable, and, for some, initially downright painful. This improves as you have further sessions. First appointments usually last 60-90 minutes, and subsequent ones 30-60 minutes.

A typical course of treatment for something like non-ovulation would be an hour's reflexology session each week for six weeks, followed by monthly top-ups. Apart from the potential physical effects on hormone levels, reflexology also offers emotional support to couples experiencing fertility problems or treatments. If a woman is being treated, her partner could benefit from some sessions too, to help deal with any stress he may be experiencing.

Who says it works?

Various studies suggest that reflexology may be effective for certain types of fertility problem. One example is the work of Devon-based reflexologist Jane Holt, who has achieved some very encouraging results during a pilot study between 1998 and 1999. During this study she treated 23 women who had difficulty becoming pregnant. All had different reasons for infertility, ranging from polycystic ovaries to recurrent miscarriage and non-ovulation, despite taking fertility drugs. Following reflexology treatment, nearly half (43%) became pregnant within the year, half of them within the first six months. At the time of writing she is conducting a randomized controlled clinical trial on 150 women with the IVF Unit of Devon's Derriford Hospital, using reflexology to treat women who were not ovulating. Their hormone levels are also being carefully measured throughout the trial to see precisely how much difference the therapy can make in measurable biochemical terms.

Another trial carried out in 1990 in Denmark involved 108 women who had all been trying for a baby without any success for an average of six and a half years. Of those who stayed with the trial and had the recommended 16 reflexology sessions over seven to eight months, one in seven became pregnant within the first six months of treatment (a result comparable to the lower success ranges of IVF).

What could a reflexologist do to help me?

A therapist might work on:

- The *Solar Plexus* area in the centre of the sole of the foot to encourage relaxation and help reduce stress.

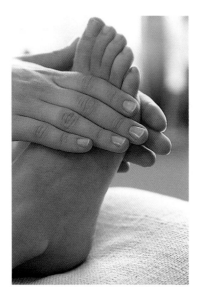

BELOW A therapist holds her patient's feet gently, part of the way through a reflexology treatment.

TIP
Always drink a couple of glasses of pure spring-water after a treatment. Reflexology enhances the circulation and nerve supply to all organs and may encourage the body to release toxins it has been storing. This could make you feel sick or headachy for a day or so, but drinking lots of water will help the kidneys flush these waste products out of your body and reduce the length of a treatment hangover, possibly even preventing it altogether.

- The *Uterine* area (mid-way between ankle bone and heel tip).
- The area corresponding to the *Fallopian tubes and Vas Deferens tubes*, found on the front on the ankle, to help relieve any energy obstructions.
- The *Hypothalamus and Pituitary gland* reflex points underneath each big toe halfway down. These are important for hormonal balance (hypothalamus) and for stimulating production of the egg-ripening hormones to encourage ovulation (pituitary).
- Points corresponding to the *Ovaries and Testes* on the outer edge of the heel, partway up towards the ankle bone.

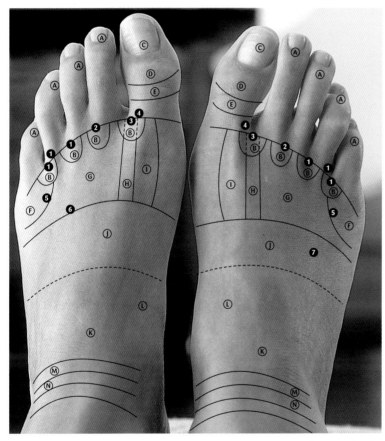

HOW LONG BEFORE I START TO FEEL BETTER?
Some people may feel benefits right away, especially from a de-stressing point of view, but the effect is usually cumulative. Depending on the problem, most therapists would treat for 5–8 sessions to begin with, gradually increasing the intervals as you begin to get better.

Some people find they react quite strongly to their first reflexology treatments. For instance, a problem may initially flare up. There may be changes in the workings of your bowels and the amount of urine you pass, or you may notice more vaginal discharge than usual or an alteration in your menstrual cycle. This is called the healing crises (as with the 'aggravation' that can briefly result from the right homeopathic remedy), but as the body starts to recover this is often when you see the most dramatic improvements.

LEFT In reflexology theory, every part of the body and every organ is reflected in very precise areas on the feet (on the tops as shown, but also on the bottom and sides, and also on the hands). This is the 'map' that shows the landscape of the tops of the feet.

GENERAL REFLEX AREAS

- (A) Head and sinuses
- (B) Submandibular and occipital lymphatics
- (C) Hair
- (D) Face
- (E) Jaw
- (F) Axillary glands
- (G) Chest, glands and lymphatics
- (H) Oesophagus, trachea and bronchials
- (I) Sternum
- (J) Upper abdominal, muscles and lymphatics
- (K) Lower abdominal
- (L) Waist
- (M) Groin and pelvic lymphatics
- (N) Fallopians/vas deferens

STRONG REFLEX POINTS

- ❶ Ear
- ❷ Eye
- ❸ Parathyroid
- ❹ Thyroid
- ❺ Shoulder
- ❻ Heart
- ❼ Gall bladder

Hypnotherapy

What is it?

There is no single, universally agreed definition of hypnotherapy. Yet it could be described as a form of psychotherapy involving deep relaxation, which helps people use the power of their own minds to change unwanted or negative thought and behaviour patterns.

Because the link between mind and body can be so strong, hypnotherapy seems to work best for problems which probably have an important psychological component, such as PMS, sleep disorders, eczema, irritable bowel syndrome and cigarette addiction. It can also be very helpful as a method of pain control.

Research in maternity units in Wales and Scotland has shown that hypnotherapy can reduce the amount of drug pain relief women need in childbirth and can shorten their labours by up to a third. American clinical trials showed it reduced pain perception markedly for patients who had surface burns covering up to 60% of their bodies. Yet hypnotherapy also appears to be successful for some thoroughly prosaic conditions which you would have thought would be immune from the mind's control – such as warts. One American study carried out in 1992 even found that hypnotherapy apparently cured verrucas in 80% of the participants in the trial.

ABOVE Hypnotherapists believe that the mind has several different levels of awareness. Under hypnosis the conscious or rational mind we use when wide awake is bypassed temporarily, allowing the subconscious part (which controls mental and physical functions) to become receptive to positive suggestion.

Can it help fertility problems?

The research available on hypnotherapy and fertility is quite fragmented, and often appears in medical journals in the form of single case studies of individual patients. Yet there is enough of it to suggest that hypnotherapy can have an effect on fertility problems. This may be because, like visualization, Autogenic Training (AT) and relaxation techniques work by harnessing the power of your own mind to work for you, rather than against you.

Italian research by Alexander Chigbugh in 1975 reviewing all the published literature he could find suggests 'psychological factors can not only inhibit ovulation, but also prevent sperm and egg meeting up by altering the pH of the vagina, producing spasms in part of the cervix (a powerfully muscular area) and also spasm in the Fallopian tubes which would prevent the egg getting down it and into the womb to implant.'

In fact, clinical work has been done on how emotional states can produce change in the body organs and tissues for decades. Some of the earliest investigations connected with gynaecological conditions and fertility were carried out back in 1965 at Stobhill General Hospital in Glasgow, Scotland. The unit looked at cases where hypnotherapy was used to treat bleeding from the womb that was not due to periods (often due to lesions, or sometimes to pre-cancerous conditions), period problems, and eight cases of infertility. It found results that were 'in general, satisfactory'.

Four particular case studies reported in 1989 in the UK on different women also make interesting reading. All of the subjects had been struggling against infertility for up to six years, and were given six hypnotherapy sessions each. One became pregnant within five weeks of treatment, having been trying to conceive for four years. This startled both therapist and patient because the woman had actually come for help in stopping biting her nails. She did so, but was also delighted to give birth to a healthy boy baby 40 weeks later. Another became pregnant six months after the last session, and yet another conceived during the course of hypnotherapy but, sadly, did miscarry at ten weeks. The last woman became pregnant five weeks after she had her final hypnotherapy session.

Another study, again carried out at the Stobhill Hospital, looked at the use of hypnotherapy to help women who could not conceive, and who also found intercourse painful. All eight participants conceived within 14 months of completing their hypnotherapy sessions, several quite quickly. They also reported that intercourse had become less painful for them.

Apart from helping to prime your body for conception, hypnotherapy may also have other major benefits which may help support both you and your partner if you are trying for a baby:

- It may help either one or both partners cope with any stress that they may be feeling. Stress can have substantial, measurable physiological effects on the sperm quality, egg quality and ripening, both sexes' structural reproductive systems and the hormones that regulate them (see Stress and infertility, page 59).
- It may help you think about whether you have any subconscious emotional blocks, which could be preventing conception. These could be anything from family pressure and financial worries, or concerns about how your partner will react to a new baby and to you in the role of a mother, to past miscarriages, abortions or even sexual abuse and violent relationships. Some women also find they have subconscious but negative or worrying thoughts about pregnancy and childbirth itself.

Autogenic Training (AT)

This is one of the most consistently researched stress-relieving techniques there is. It has been likened to self-hypnosis – which is why it appears in this section – but is really closer to meditation. It is used for all types of stress-related problem.

AT is said to work by enabling you to control your autonomic nervous system, switching it from sympathetic control (which reacts to stress) to parasympathetic control (which encourages rest and relaxation) at will.

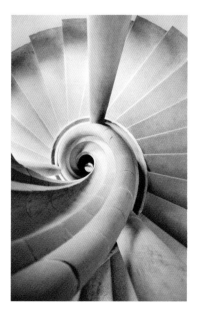

BELOW A therapist may use the image of a descending flight of stairs that you walk down, counting from step one to ten, to help bring about a relaxed but focused state of mind.

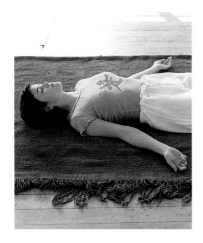

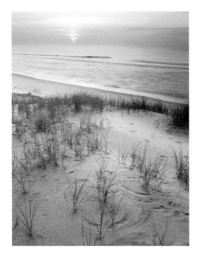

TOP A hypnotherapist would usually teach you simple forms of self-hypnosis - generally involving deep relaxation, plus affirmations and positive imagery - to reinforce the treatment when you are at home. Many people like to do this lying down comfortably, others prefer to sit.

ABOVE During hypnosis the therapist would ask you to imagine yourself in a calm and beautiful place where you felt both happy and completely safe. Many people choose a soothing natural scenario like this one.

Taught individually or in groups of about ten people at a time, the training sessions last 8-10 weeks, with one instruction session a week and daily practice in between. The first part of the course involves mastering the six standard autogenic exercises, which are eventually run together as a continuous routine lasting 20-30 minutes. They are simple and effective, focusing on controlling your breathing, heart rate, body temperature, muscle tension and so on.

You are taught to make your limbs feel heavy and warm, to give yourself a calm, regular heartbeat, regular breathing, warmth in the abdomen and solar plexus, and a feeling of coolness on your forehead. At the end of these six exercises there is a 'quiet space' when you are completely relaxed, which can be used to introduce an affirmation. An affirmation is a reassurance or instruction that you give to yourself, and 'plant' in your own mind when it is at its most receptive. It could be 'I will sleep well tonight and wake refreshed', 'I will remain calm throughout my medical tests tomorrow' or 'I can, and will, become pregnant'.

The second group of exercises focuses on releasing emotional or physical tension in direct ways like punching pillows, crying or shouting. Over the weeks you will build up a battery of techniques to help you cope with stress.

What could a hypnotherapist do to help me?

During hypnotherapy you are neither asleep nor powerless but in a different state of consciousness, similar to when you are just about to fall asleep. You are deeply relaxed, your mind is receptive to change and suggestion, you can concentrate intensely - yet you cannot be made to do or say anything you do not wish to do. You are still in control of your own behaviour, despite scare stories which occasionally appear in the media. A professionally trained and reputable therapist merely gives you suggestions, which you yourself decide whether you wish to follow or not.

POSITIVE THOUGHTS
The subconscious mind will believe almost anything you tell it. Hypnotherapy utilizes this by replacing negative beliefs with positive ones.

Ideas and feelings that are blocking conception can, with the patient's informed cooperation, be re-framed during hypnotherapy and replaced with far more positive impressions. Fears and past distress can be gently acknowledged, respected and worked through.

What does treatment involve?

The first session is usually an assessment and can last 60-90 minutes. It covers why you have come to see the therapist, your medical/personal history and any questions you have about hypnotherapy.

The hypnotherapist may induce hypnosis in a first session if there is time. Different therapists use different techniques. These are far less dramatic than most of us imagine, and involve lying back comfortably on a couch or reclining chair while the hypnotherapist literally talks you gently into a deeply relaxed state.

He or she may encourage you to use gentle deep breathing techniques, and also to imagine yourself descending a stairway of ten steps, encouraging you to become more deeply relaxed at each step you take downwards until you find yourself in a calm place of your own choosing where you feel safe and happy. Many people at this point like to imagine they are looking at a beautiful outdoors scene, perhaps on a favourite deserted sunny beach, by a calm lake, or lying in a hammock under a tree on holiday.

The therapist may then talk you slowly through your reproductive system, getting you to imagine each part of it in turn as whole and healthy; then begin to talk about fertilization. You may be reminded that you are fertile, that there is nothing stopping you from creating a pregnancy of your own. If you are a woman, you may be helped to visualize a ripe egg being ovulated, 'see' it in your mind's eye being stroked gently down the tubes by the delicate, tentacle-like cilia. You may then be encouraged to imagine the fertilized egg burrowing into the plush, welcoming, soft womb lining that your body has made ready for it; and then to see it implanting there safely and securely.

If you are a man, the therapist might encourage you to imagine how strong, fast, healthy and well-formed your sperm are; how plentiful they are in number; and to visualize them racing towards, breaking into and fertilizing an egg.

To bring you out of light hypnosis, your therapist will help you count yourself slowly back up the ten stairs and into full consciousness. Afterwards, most people feel very peaceful and relaxed as if waking from a good nap, and find they yawn and stretch a little.

A typical course of hypnotherapy will last anything from two to eight sessions, depending on the issues or problems you uncover. A good therapist would also probably teach you how to put yourself into light self-hypnosis. This reduces any potential dependence upon them, and also enables you to carry on with any fertility and pregnancy-enhancing work at home, in your own time.

VISUALIZATION
Some people describe visualization as being like watching a film in their heads, in which they themselves can appear at will.

ALWAYS
- Talk to the hypnotherapist over the phone first. Discuss the reason why you want to see them and give them a little background, rather than just briefly making an appointment.
- Ask what experience they have in helping with fertility issues.
- Trust your instincts when you meet them. If you are not quite comfortable with them (whether or not you can put your finger on the reason), simply pay for the session but say you need to go away and think about it further before having hypnosis.

Relaxation and Visualization

What is it?

Relaxation and visualization (R&V) are two separate disciplines, though they are often used together as a single therapy. At their simplest level:

- **Relaxation is a straightforward physical technique that is used to combat stress.**
- **Visualization is the conscious use of your imagination to create positive images which can help heal or change aspects of your life, including your health. Literally, 'seeing' yourself better.**

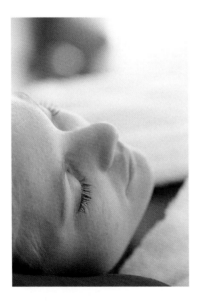

BELOW Visualization is a technique which harnesses the enormous power of your own imagination to help you cope with stress, fulfil your potential and enhance your body's natural ability to work healthily and to heal itself.

WORKING TOGETHER
What your mind does, it can also undo. Techniques such as relaxation or visualization can encourage your body to work for you rather than against you.

Modern medicine has only recently accepted the fact that a person's mind and body work as an integrated unit, though this is a belief long held by holistic and complementary health practitioners and Eastern philosophers. It took the dawning of the new sciences of psycho-neuro-biology (the effect of the mind on the corporal body) and psycho-neuroimmunology (how the mind affects the immune system) to convince orthodox doctors that the mind has power to affect the body physically, and vice versa.

Many women who are experiencing fertility problems, such as miscarriage or inability to conceive, have said that they feel that their bodies are letting them down, or even working against them. As one said in *The Observer* magazine (22 April 2001): 'My reproductive system was playing lots of nasty tricks on me and I didn't trust it an inch'.

Anyone who suspects that stress may be a factor in their fertility problems can reduce its effects if they use relaxation techniques regularly. Published clinical data has repeatedly shown that severe or prolonged stress can play havoc with both men's and women's fertility (see Stress and infertility, page 59). This is an instinctive and completely reasonable response to feeling threatened. Animals find it harder to reproduce if they don't feel safe and comfortable (witness the mating pairs who refuse to breed in the captivity of zoos under the public eye) and so do we.

Disciplines including hypnotherapy, Autogenic Training, yoga and meditation, all of which involve relaxation and visualization, have been used successfully in hospital units and clinical trials to combat many different types of health problem, from heart disorders and inflammatory bowel disease to sleep dysfunction and headaches. Relaxation and visualization techniques are straightforward to learn from a qualified practitioner. Yet it is also possible to learn simple techniques without a teacher's help, in your own home. They can help you dissolve and let go of everyday stresses, and can also be used to cope with very specific situations such as having clinically assisted conception treatments, like IVF.

Relaxation

Relaxation is not just a matter of curling up in front of the TV with a glass of wine. This feels good, but you are still being bombarded with outside stimuli – sounds and images from the TV, the kick of the wine – and your body is probably still in a sitting position rather than lying flat out comfortably. More to the point, you are not letting go of anything which may have wound you up during the day, such as the after-effects of commuting to work, queueing in a supermarket, work pressure and the continual assault on the senses that is inner-city living if you live in a major town.

'Real' therapeutic relaxation is a healing process that focuses all your attention on calming your mind and your body, and is something of an acquired skill. This skill gets easier quickly with practice and it need not take long either. Ten minutes at the end of the day can make a real difference to how you are feeling and coping.

Relaxation works on your physical body. It rebalances the sympathetic and parasympathetic parts of the autonomic nervous system. The sympathetic system is in charge of all the vital functions which you perform involuntarily without having to think about them – your heartbeat, your breathing rate, your adrenaline-fuelled 'fight or flight' response. You can teach yourself to relax 'lightly' using regulated breathing and muscular techniques without needing to be shown how by a tutor.

However, if you would like to learn deep relaxation techniques, you will need to be taught by a professionally trained therapist or tutor. These techniques involve disciplines such as hypnotherapy (you can be taught simple self-hypnosis), meditation (such as Transcendental Meditation), Autogenic Training (see page 101) and chakra work. These can induce a trance-like state, and their effects are more profound and last longer than those of the briefer relaxation techniques which can be used for coping with everyday stress.

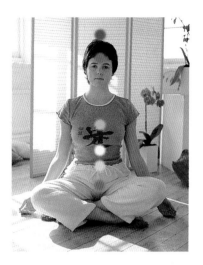

ABOVE Some people use chakra work as part of visualization for mental and physical health. According to esoteric teachings (including yoga, and Eastern medicine) the seven chakras are the spiritual energy centres of the body. Each has a different colour and set of functions associated with it.

Visualization

Your brain is divided into two hemispheres. The right side relates to creativity, emotion and imagination. The left is in charge of logical thought and reason. Most of the time we are using the left – to work, study and carry out routine tasks. Visualization encourages right brain activity. It uses the images it creates to over-write any destructive effects created by the left side. So if you can give your mind a strong, positive image (provided it is theoretically attainable and one you can believe in) it will accept that instead of a negative one it is holding. A therapist will usually teach you visualization using positive guided imagery, talking you through a scenario.

A BRIEF NOTE OF CAUTION

Visualizations involving grass or flowers are evocative, calming and beautiful to imagine but they have also been known to trigger off an asthma or allergy attack in people who are sensitive to these plants.

TOGETHER THEY'RE STRONGER
Relaxation is beneficial and valuable when it is used alone. However, its effects are even more powerful if you combine them with mental techniques, such as visualization.

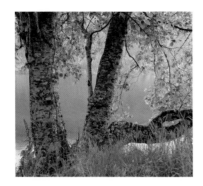

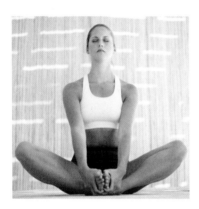

TOP Using other senses in your mind (apart from 'sight') to create a visualization scenario in your head will make it more powerful. For instance, try to 'hear' in your mind the lapping of calm waters, the rustle of fresh leaves, 'feel' the softness of new grass under your bare feet.

ABOVE This meditation or visualization position is good for helping to keep your back comfortably straight, and is an alternative to the traditional yoga half-lotus position. If neither feels right, just sit on a chair with a supportive back or lie down, as the idea is to feel relaxed and comfortable.

Someone with respiration difficulties such as asthma may also experience initial problems if asked to focus on their breathing, though relaxation and visualization is successfully used to treat asthma too.

People with heart disorders may initially become more aware of their heartbeat slowing, and find this disconcerting. Most methods do involve breathing techniques (doing so more slowly and deeply) and a slowing down of the heart rate. If you have concerns about your health or breathing consult a professional therapist.

Relaxation and visualization techniques

There are four broad categories of relaxation technique. Regulated breathing plays an important part in many of them. Visualization plays a part in most of them.

TENSE-RELEASE

Tensing up then releasing muscle groups is the basis of many different types of relaxation technique. It has been used for many years in midwifery, yoga and medicine and it is one of the most common methods that therapists now teach. The idea is to tense up your muscles then release them again, feeling as you do so the mental and physical 'letting go' that accompanies this movement. This is often accompanied by breathing *in* as you tense up, then breathing or blowing air *out* again as you let go. The shoulder shrug to calm tense neck and shoulder muscles is one you have probably done many times yourself.

You could strengthen the effect of the *tense-release* method by adding a simple visualization. Imagine that as you breathe air in you are also breathing in peace and calm. Then imagine the tension flowing out of you as you breathe out. It could be in the form of:

- A wave, rolling down the part of your body you are concentrating on (e.g. shoulders) and breaking out beyond where your body ends, as if on a shore.
- Excess heat radiating away from the area you are concentrating on.
- A particular colour washing through this part of your body, and out again into the surrounding air, taking your tension with it.

A therapist would probably 'talk' you all around your body encouraging you to tense and relax every part in turn, beginning with an arm or a leg.

PASSIVE MUSCLE RELAXATION

You need to be familiar with your muscle groups for this one but, once you are, it's quicker than the tense-release method and you can do it anywhere. The idea is similar to tense-release except that instead of tensing a muscle group or clenching it you concentrate upon it, acknowledge the tension is there and release it mentally. A therapist might suggest you imagine a warm, slow wave of relaxation washing through those muscles, lengthening and expanding them.

VISUALIZATION

Visualization involves using the power of your mind instead of your muscles. You could:

- See yourself as you want to be, in your mind's eye. A professional athlete might prepare for a sporting event by visualizing herself winning before entering a race. A woman who wants to become pregnant might regularly visualize her ripe egg being released, fertilized, then implanting itself in her womb safely – and growing into a healthy baby which she is holding in her arms at the end.
- See yourself in a special, safe imaginary place. When you are completely relaxed and lying back with your eyes closed, the therapist suggests that you choose a place that is beautiful and calm, a place where you want to be. It could be a secret garden entered by a hidden gate, a tropical island, a deserted sunny beach, a soft grassy bank under a willow tree by a green river, even a favourite armchair by the fire in a beloved childhood home.

The therapist will encourage you to imagine you are using your senses to actually explore your special place, hearing birds or waves, seeing the colours of the flowers or the sea, feeling the grass or sand under your bare feet. You will be led in the exercise and gently given suggestions and guidance, but the beauty of visualization is that you can put what you like into your special place because it is yours, and no one else's. Choose what works best for you.

Your mind is now totally relaxed, and a relaxed mind is receptive to anything you wish to give it. You can use this stage to give yourself an affirmation. An affirmation is a powerful, positive personal message or statement. It could be 'I will win that race tomorrow', or 'I will sleep well and deeply tonight' or 'I am healthy, fertile and am going to get pregnant.' What would yours be?

DEEP TECHNIQUES

Deep techniques include Autogenic Training, meditation, chakra work and hypnotherapy. These methods can be immensely effective but they take longer to learn because they are more complicated than simple relaxation and visualization.

They also need to be taught by a professional practitioner, for several reasons. For one, they may lower your blood pressure considerably. Also, some people find that, a little way into their training, tension, distress, major fears or deep-rooted anxieties that they have been strenuously suppressing (perhaps for many years) can come to the surface. If this happens to you, you may be glad of a trained therapist to help you work through them.

However, once you have learned these techniques, you've got them for life and you can use them whenever you need to. They become easier and more effective every time you practise them if you are able to do so regularly (aim for three times a week; more is even better).

VERY EASY FIVE-MINUTE RELAXATION

- Lie on your back on the floor or on a bed. Make sure your body is straight, chin tucked in. Hands should be by your sides, palms upwards. Legs slightly apart and bent a little at the knee, if this is more comfortable.
- Breathe in steadily and gently for a count of six. Hold for six. Breathe out for six. Repeat six times.
- Let go of tension. Starting at your head and neck let stiffness and tension flow out of your body. Work down to your shoulders. Now your arms. Your chest, back, tummy, hips. Move on to your legs and finally feet, all the way to your toes.
- To complete, on the next in-breath bring your arms up over your head and stretch out your whole body. Bring your arms back down to your sides as you breathe out again. Repeat twice. Then lie still and relax for a few moments.
- Now roll gently over onto your side, and sit up.

Feng Shui

Feng Shui (pronounced 'fong shway') means *wind and water* in Chinese. It refers to the way in which the earth's geography of hills, mountains, rivers, seas and valleys is shaped by the continuous interaction of these two most powerful forces of nature.

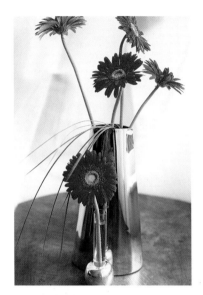

ABOVE Bright red or purple flowers are seen as very auspicious in all the classical Feng Shui texts.

What is it?

Feng Shui is the art – and the science – of creating harmony and balance in your own environment. Its practitioners and clients say that if it's done correctly it can have a powerfully positive effect on every single aspect of your life, from romance and family life to business and health. Its laws provide rules for choosing between good and problematic locations, positioning homes and designing room layouts in ways that may enhance the quality of their owners' lives dramatically.

> 'In Chinese cultures where family life and honour are very strong, good Feng Shui is also seen as helping husbands and wives beget many good and loving children who will bring honour to the family name.'
> *Lillian Too, former Managing Director of Grindlays Dao Heng Bank in Hong Kong, and international authority on Feng Shui*

However, bad Feng Shui is thought to bring about illness, accidents, financial problems and general bad luck.

Many traditional cultures have some Feng Shui-like systems of their own but the most sophisticated and comprehensive has been developed in China. The term first appeared in military texts back in AD900 to set guidelines for the safe deployment of soldiers, but the basis of those guidelines may date back many hundreds, or even thousands, of years earlier. Feng Shui is now enjoying a spectacular revival in its countries of origin, and over the last five years it has also been taken increasingly seriously in the West.

Part of the appeal of Feng Shui is that it has a foot in two camps, one in the basic principles of good design and common sense, the other in a more spiritual and traditional set of principles. The combination is attracting Westerners who are becoming used to certain Eastern systems of medicine and thought, such as acupuncture and Ayurvedic medicine, and who are increasingly interested in complementary, holistic approaches to life's challenges, whether they be in body or mind.

How does it work?

Feng Shui uses the design of your surroundings as a channelling or controlling force in order to make the most of 'good' or positive natural energies, and deflect or minimize the effects of any negative ones.

More modern practitioners, especially if they are involved in design and management consultancy, might offer a psychology-based explanation. They believe that you can adjust your environment so that it stimulates your subconscious, and therefore encourages your actions to be in harmony with the things you want to bring about.

A Westerner or someone who had never heard of Feng Shui might say a place with good Feng Shui would have 'a good atmosphere'; that it was a place they were comfortable and happy to spend time in.

NEGATIVE ENERGIES

Traditional Feng Shui refers to 'poison arrows' – negative energy emitted or caused by sharp pointed objects or structures, and producing what the Chinese call 'killing breath' (negative energy). Causes of poison arrows include sharp room corners, furniture corners, heavy shelving above your bedhead and old-fashioned exposed ceiling beams. A modern Feng Shui practitioner may refer to these, less esoterically, as threatening or unharmonious design features.

Also included in the poison arrow list are any sharp outside structures, which may channel or direct negative energy into your home. These include sharply pointed angles on house roofs opposite where you live, a single tall thin tree, a church spire, a high tower or chimney, a protruding corner, a straight road directly opposite and leading to or from your front door (as in a T-junction or even a dead straight garden path), or any large overhanging or overshadowing object.

POSITIVE ENERGY

The design of a space is vitally important so that positive chi (energy) can flow through it unhindered by obstacles in its path, yet not slip through so fast that it doesn't linger long enough to do any good.

Factors which can create a good steady flow of positive or auspicious energy include curves (walls, furniture, the garden path, garden flowerbeds), well-placed healthy plants, wind-chimes and mobiles, carefully sited mirrors, uplighters creating soft light, daylight, refracting prisms, glass globes and crystals. Stabilizers include heavy natural rocks, stones or points.

The location of doors, windows and main furniture pieces – especially your bed – can all create excellent Feng Shui energy. A good balance in your rooms, home and office environments is also important – getting the ratio between energizing and stimulating factors (e.g. strong colours, bold pictures, lots of bright daylight) which the Chinese call yang, and the soothing, low-key factors which are known as yin.

Modern Feng Shui

The more modern systems of Feng Shui are based on principles derived from mathematics, the ancient Chinese *I Ching* (*Book of Changes*) and the main points of the compass (N, NE, SW and so on). There are two main systems. The first uses a device called a Pa Gua or Ba-Gua. This is

---

DIY IMITATIONS

Be wary of DIY Feng Shui from a book. Books are helpful for the background and general principles but the author hasn't checked out *your* home or met you. Just as a book on homeopathy can give you a lot of background and some good tips, a book on Feng Shui can do the same. However, you won't get anywhere near the results that seeing a professional in person would provide.

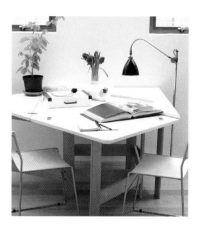

ABOVE Feng Shui is being used increasingly in Western working environments to improve luck, good health at work and productivity – whether they are a quiet corner at home, or a huge multi-story bank.

IMPORTANT

Check your front door is not being hit by a poison arrow from outside your home. Feng Shui teaching says this can bring considerable ill fortune. If it is, it may often be deflected by a well-placed Pa Gua mirror hung on the front door to send the negative energy back to its source.

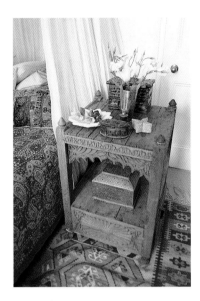

ABOVE Antiques and second-hand goods – especially beds – are considered bad Feng Shui since you don't know the luck of the people who owned them before.

an octagonal instrument designed around the numbers one to nine, giving nine different directions. Each of the eight sides features a different symbolic trigram or hexagram pattern from the *I Ching*, and there is a yin/yang sign in its centre in position no. 9. The Pa Gua system has been adapted to modern living for people who live in flats and terraces; their reference point for allocating their home's personal 'points of the compass' is their own front door, rather than the usual magnetic north.

Each of the nine directions is associated with different things, and these include:

- A particular point of the compass
- A basic personality or character type based upon your date of birth (a little like Western astrology)
- The body's main organs
- Colours
- One of the five traditional Chinese environmental elements – fire, earth, metal, water and wood, and their type (e.g. 'small wood', 'big metal' and so on)
- The important main areas of a person's life, including the home, family relationships, wealth and health.

A practitioner will work out a place's Feng Shui, whether it is a single room or a 50-floor office block, using the Pa Gua and a design layout of the place.

The other system of Feng Shui does not use a Pa Gua device, but works with the five different traditional Chinese elements – wood, earth, fire, water and metal. According to the laws of Feng Shui, a good balanced environment is one where some of the characteristics of each of those five elements is present in some form or another in fairly even proportions. The proportions can be adjusted in each home or workplace, according to what each of the rooms, or even the different areas within a single room, is to be used for.

Five steps to Feng Shui

1 *De-clutter*: The first step to creating harmony and a good energy flow throughout your home is to get rid of any clutter and rubbish *right away*. Do a tour of your home, making your own personal clutter/rubbish list room by room. Anything which is no longer (a) used regularly (b) good to look at (c) giving you pleasure, should be thrown out.
2 *Mend* anything that's broken and is worth repairing (furniture that is coming unglued, blown lightbulbs, stopped clocks and cracked windowpanes).
3 *Complete* projects (e.g. paint that half-done sitting room, finish building that garden wall, resolve that longstanding argument with family, friends or neighbours). These are major obstructions to

MIRROR, MIRROR ...
Never have big mirrors in the bedroom that either face you as you get up or reflect you in bed. It suggests the intrusion of third parties, and is said to encourage trouble between husband and wife, or infidelity.

harmony and your own personal progress. Once out of the way, this boosts a positive feeling of moving forward – and 'getting there' which is invaluable psychologically.

4 *Look and think*: What is in my space? How is it affecting me? The place where you sleep is of paramount importance. Good Feng Shui in your bedroom is vital to good sex, a happy romantic relationship with a partner, conception, pregnancy and the general good luck of your entire household.

5 *Now make changes*. The advice you get may vary depending on which Feng Shui practitioner you talk to. Go with what feels right and rings a bell with you.

FENG SHUI IN THE BEDROOM

- Use warm, soft colours* to create a haven of safety and cosiness in your bedroom. Try to choose your bedroom so it gets the morning sun and stimulates your pituitary glands (also important for orchestrating the sex hormones).
- Have pictures of babies and some, perhaps a couple of, cuddly toys around to work on your subconscious.
- Remove any objects or pictures which have any negative associations for you.
- Ensure the bed faces the door (though not directly opposite it) and backs onto a wall for a feeling of safety.
- Do not have shelves above your bedhead.
- Do not have anything pointed (e.g. a pretty ethnic triangular silk lampshade) hanging down over the bed.

Simon Brown, UK Feng Shui 'consultant to the stars', has the following further suggestions:

- Sleep so the top of your head points northwards, as northern chi energy is especially helpful to conception.
- Decorate your room in cream colours, and have pure cream-coloured bed-linen (*see how different practitioners can offer very different ideas?).
- Place a crystal in the northern part of your home to activate northern chi energy still further.
- Wear pure cotton clothing to decrease static generated by synthetic materials.

The two most important points are to keep your bedroom, and especially your Relationship Corner, clean, tidy and clutter-free, *and to reserve your bedroom exclusively for sleeping and sex.* Never, ever take work there or allow a TV in this room.

FOR STIMULATING SEXUALITY AND ROMANCE

Feng Shui lore suggests that you work on your Relationship Corner. That's the area on the right end of the wall that is opposite the door. Arrange the following items there:

- Purple candles.
- A permanent small vase of fresh, red or deep pink flowers. Just two beautiful blooms will do if you don't want too obtrusive a display. Go for sensual-looking flowers like lilies or peonies.
- An erotic picture which you both like.

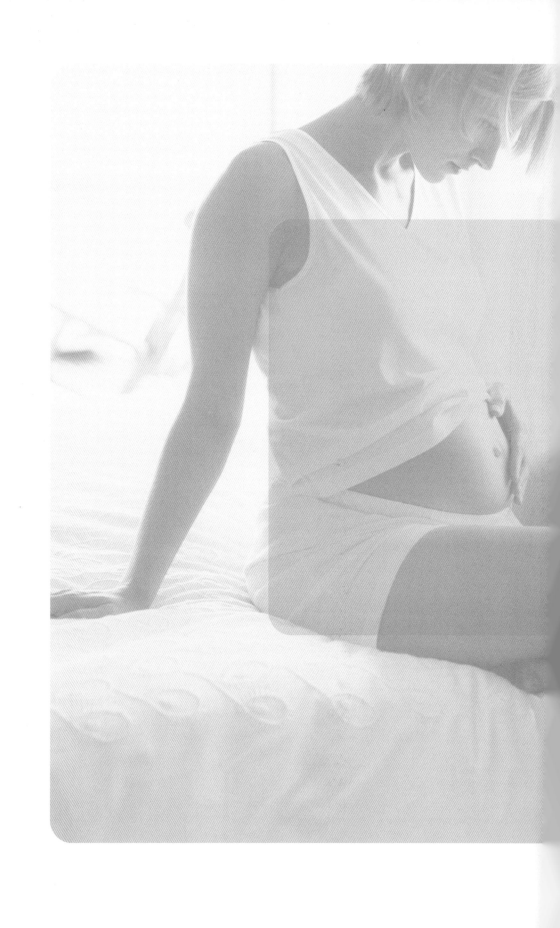

The Medical Side of Fertility Treatment

This section offers an overview of the most common reasons for fertility problems, the medical investigations that can pin-point them, and the orthodox clinical treatments that can help.

The number of people seeking support and medical help because they cannot get pregnant has rocketed by 55% just in the last five years, even though statistically couples who want to get pregnant have generally been doing so more quickly over the past ten years than in previous decades.

Every year, in the UK alone, one in six couples experiences a fertility problem and 27,000 couples have fertility treatment. Around 1 in 80 babies is now born this way in the UK, and in Denmark the figure is nearer to 1 in 40.

There is a lot of hope, joy and distress hidden in those bald little statistics. They also show that, if you do find you need any infertility treatment, you are certainly not alone.

Medical infertility treatments are usually expensive, most are invasive, and nearly all are stressful. They are the last thing to go for, not the first. Yet the technology and clinical skill involved in them are at their most impressive level ever. And their success rates have never been higher.

Overall, around half the people having fertility treatments of different sorts will have a baby of their own by the end of it. In fact, whether you are using a good preconception care programme, having medical fertility treatments, or both, the chances of having the baby you long for are better than they have ever been before.

What Can Cause Fertility Problems in Women?

Common reasons for not getting pregnant

Ovulation is the release of a ripe egg from an ovary. Ovaries come in matched pairs that lie snugly on either side of the womb. Each month during a woman's fertile years one ovary releases a ripened egg into the nearest Fallopian tube. If no egg is released there will be no pregnancy. It is estimated that for around a quarter of couples having difficulty conceiving, the cause is related to ovulation.

OVULATION PROBLEMS

General health problems can disturb the balance between a woman's pituitary, hypothalamus and ovaries, so she either does not ovulate at all, or does so erratically. Weight loss, being overweight, stress and distress, thyroid problems and excessive exercise can have the same effect. Smoking may lower oestrogen levels and have a knock-on effect on luteinizing hormone (LH), the hormone responsible for ripening the egg. This is why smoking affects your chances of becoming pregnant.

Endometriosis occurring around the ovaries and polycystic ovary syndrome (see page 115) may also stop the release of eggs. Some types of hormonal contraception can delay the return of your natural ovulation patterns (see What contraception?, page 44). Sometimes it is the pituitary gland itself which is at fault and failing to send out the right hormonal signals for egg ripening and release, perhaps because it is damaged or even (very rarely) because of a benign tumour there.

Once a woman has reached the menopause she will no longer ovulate. Sometimes the menopause happens prematurely, before the age of 40. Doctors cannot always find a reason for a premature menopause, though it is known to run in families. Some women's bodies make 'auto-antibodies', which stop their ovaries working, and a few have had a viral infection, which has attacked and damaged the area. Very occasionally in cases of premature menopause ovaries will start working again without treatment.

There is also a condition called resistant ovary syndrome, where the ovaries become increasingly immune to the action of the FSH and LH hormones, which stimulate egg ripening.

A doctor can test your hormone levels with blood tests. But, because levels vary throughout the menstrual cycle anyway, it is important that your physician checks with you as to whereabouts in your cycle you are and when you expect to have your period.

BLOCKED FALLOPIAN TUBES

This is a very common cause of fertility problems. There are many reasons why tubes can become blocked, and one of the commonest is a previous infection in the pelvis. This can produce internal scarring called

BELOW This is an image from a hysterosalpinogram of a woman's abdomen. The X-ray-sensitive dye shows that the right Fallopian tube is enlarged, but the left one is not showing up at all. This suggests the latter is blocked where the tube joins the womb, since the dye was unable to flow into it.

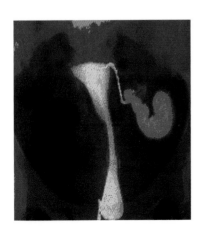

adhesions, which look like cobwebs between the pelvic organs. They can sometimes gum up the finger-like ends of the tubes (the fimbriae) so the egg cannot enter, or may even cover the ovaries themselves like biological clingfilm. Adhesions may be caused by infections from a previous miscarriage, abortion, an infection from a contraceptive IUD or a sexually transmitted disease (especially chlamydia), appendicitis, abdominal surgery or endometriosis.

The two main tests to check on the health of your Fallopian tubes are a hysterosalpinogram (HSG) and a laparoscopy. The former involves injecting fluid through the neck of your womb (cervix) and using X-rays to follow its flow through the womb and up into your tubes. This will show where any blockages, polyps or adhesions are. A laparoscopy involves threading a fine telescope into your abdomen under general anaesthetic, so the surgeon can take a close careful look at your ovaries, womb and tubes. Actual treatment (surgically removing any areas of endometriosis or adhesions found) can also be done at the same time as the visual check.

DELICATE TUBING

Almost one in every three cases of women's infertility is caused by damage in the delicate Fallopian tubes – no wider than a fine pin inside – which bring the ripened egg down from ovary to womb. The egg is usually fertilized in these tubes too.

POLYCYSTIC OVARY SYNDROME (POS)

Polycystic ovary syndrome is a type of ovulation disorder. Three-quarters of the women who come to a fertility clinic for help with ovulation problems have POS. The term polycystic literally means 'many cysts', which can sound a bit alarming. However, all ovaries, if they are working normally, have a few cysts. These are the follicles in which the eggs ripen. The only difference between ordinary ovaries and polycystic ovaries is that the latter are a little bigger and contain more follicles (cysts). This may or may not affect fertility.

Polycystic ovaries are not, in themselves, abnormal at all. In fact one in five women has them and only a small proportion of these will have any fertility problems. For women in whom they do cause problems, the symptoms experienced include erratic periods (sometimes no periods at all) and extra unwanted body hair. There is also a link with weight; one-third of women with polycystic ovary syndrome are overweight and their fertility can improve dramatically if they lose some.

POS can be diagnosed from its symptoms (irregular or absent periods, extra body hair), blood tests to check for hormone levels and an ultrasound scan of the ovaries.

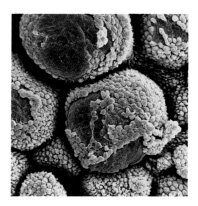

ABOVE This is a polycystic ovary (PCO) showing some ripening egg follicles bulging out against the ovary wall. However, with PCO the ovaries are reluctant to release any of those eggs. Fertility drugs may help women who are not ovulating as a result of this condition; and if you are overweight, losing some can also help.

ENDOMETRIOSIS

Endometriosis is a condition in which the cells of the womb lining (endometrium) are found in other areas of the body, usually within the pelvis. Wherever they are – in the womb wall, Fallopian tubes, ovaries, bowel, bladder and occasionally in more far-flung locations such as the lungs, heart and eyes – they will continue to respond to natural hormonal cycles, and will bleed each time the woman has a period.

It is thought that endometriosis is quite common, that it is normal to have a mild degree of the condition, and that it is only a problem if it becomes extensive or if a woman is especially sensitive to it. The

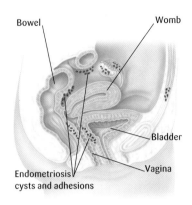

Bowel

Womb

Bladder

Vagina

Endometriosis
cysts and adhesions

ABOVE This shows some of the places where fragments of womb-lining tissue can grow, and produce endometriosis. The condition may well not affect your fertility at all, but if it does cause you problems with either your periods or with conception, there are many different treatments, both orthodox and complementary, that can help.

National Endometriosis Society (UK) suggests that there are two million women who have it in Britain. There is an unhelpful stereotype of the typical person with endometriosis – a thirty-something career woman who has delayed childbearing. In fact any woman between puberty and the menopause can develop it.

> **WANDERING WOMB LINING**
> There have even been reports of women who experienced nosebleeds when they had their period, and at least one who shed 'tears of blood' each month.

The blood produced by endometriosis has no escape route from the body, unlike the womb lining which sheds via the cervical os, and the result of this is inflammation, pain and the formation of scar tissue. If endometrial tissue forms in the ovaries it can form 'chocolate cysts' of old, dark blood.

The symptoms of endometriosis include painful or heavy periods, ovulation pain, pain before you begin your periods, pain during intercourse and pain during an internal pelvic examination.

No one is too sure what causes endometriosis. The different theories include retrograde menstruation, whereby some of your menstrual blood is thought to flow backwards up the Fallopian tubes and into your pelvis. This blood contains cells from the endometrium, which then implant themselves on your reproductive organs or in other areas (usually within the pelvis). The implanted cells can then flourish and grow into islands of displaced womb lining. Other possibilities include an immune system problem, genetic predisposition (since it can run in families) and exposure to certain environmental pollutants such as dioxin.

There is a wide range of possible treatments for this disorder which may help, though not cure it completely, ranging from drugs and laser surgery to complementary therapies (such as homeopathy, herbalism and acupuncture; see Which treatment?, page 125).

MAKING ANTIBODIES TO YOUR PARTNER'S SPERM
See section on Cervical mucus problems, page 117.

FIBROIDS
Fibroids are benign (non-cancerous) growths in, or on, the wall of the womb. They are very common indeed, and between a fifth and a third of all women are thought to have a fibroid or two of one sort or another. They can measure just a few millimetres across, or reach impressive sizes of 30–40 cm (12–15 inches), though it is unusual for them to grow this large. They may grow in several different positions in the womb. Some hang from a little stalk inside it, even outside it; some grow inside the womb's wall (intramural fibroids) or on the outside wall of the womb (sub-serous fibroids).

Fibroids are made from smooth muscle fibre, just like the rest of the womb. They tend to be more common, and cause more problems, for Afro-Caribbean and African women.

You may never know you have a fibroid because they often cause no symptoms and, as long as they are not exerting any pressure on neighbouring organs or taking up too much room, you can live with them quite happily for years.

However, they can also cause infertility. The fact you have a fibroid or fibroids does not necessarily mean you will have difficulty becoming pregnant, but there are several possible ways in which they could interfere with conception. For instance, they may alter the blood supply to the womb, they may alter the way your womb contracts, they can block the exit to the Fallopian tube or tubes, and if they are distorting the inside surface of your womb this could make it harder for a tiny fertilized embryo to implant there. Fibroids which are large enough to take up a lot of space in the uterine cavity (space inside your womb) itself by their sheer size may also increase the risk of miscarriage.

Most fibroids are diagnosed by an ultrasound scan. They can be treated with drugs to shrink them (not that successful) or removed surgically; or laser treatment can cauterize the blood vessels supplying them so that they shrink gently away.

CERVICAL MUCUS PROBLEMS

It is estimated that for 1 in 20 women experiencing fertility problems, the difficulty lies with the cervical mucus they are making. The mucus itself is made by tiny glands inside the os, the slim canal in the centre of your cervix, which leads from the vagina to the womb. It usually does a very good job of protecting the womb from any invading infections by creating a sticky barrier they cannot get through.

However, around ovulation time, the extra oestrogen your body is producing causes the mucus to become watery, clear and 'stretchy' instead, very like egg white. Sperm can swim though this and up into the womb to search out a ripe egg. This type of cervical mucus is a haven for sperm after the acidity of the vagina.

After ovulation, your body produces extra progesterone which makes the mucus thicker, sticker and scantier – again, no sperm can get through this.

There are three ways in which cervical mucus can prevent you getting pregnant. This could happen if:

- there is not enough of it to allow the sperm to move easily
- it is too thick and sticky, so sperm cannot swim through it
- it contains antibodies to your partner's sperm cells.

Tests to check for these things include the following:

- *Post-coital test (PCT)*: For a PCT, a doctor checks a small sample of your cervical mucus under a microscope between 6 and 12 hours after you and your partner have had sexual intercourse together. If the test is normal (positive) it will show live sperm swimming in the mucus sample. If the result is negative, it means that the sperm are

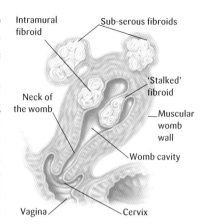

ABOVE These show the most usual places for fibroids to grow. They may be the size of a pea, an orange or larger. Fibroids often have no effect whatsoever on your fertility. If they do, surgical removal is usually successful, although they may grow again elsewhere.

BELOW Healthy cervical mucus crystallizes if it is placed on a glass lab slide into a beautiful pattern that resembles the delicate branching fronds of a young fern (see page 118).

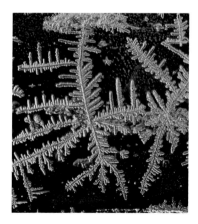

either swimming slowly and aimlessly, or that they are all dead. If this happens, your doctor should do several more PCTs over a period of a few weeks, as the test may at first be negative even though there is nothing wrong with your mucus, meaning a negative result can be a one-off.

- *Ferning*: This test involves placing a small drop of your mucus on a slide and allowing it to dry. As it does so, it should crystallize into a beautiful pattern that looks like fern leaves. The amount of branches the fern has depends on your levels of oestrogen and progesterone, so this test can also be used to check that your mucus is responding normally to your sex hormones.
- *Examination of your mucus under a microscope* with (a) some of your partner's live sperm, then (b) a sample of healthy sperm taken from a donor.

Investigations should also include checks for genital infections. Trichomoniasis for instance, can affect the cervical mucus and is straightforward to treat.

Repeated miscarriages

If you have ever miscarried, you are certainly not alone because one in every seven confirmed pregnancies doesn't last. And very early miscarriage (within 1–14 days of fertilization) is thought to happen up to three-quarters of the time, usually because the early embryo either couldn't implant in the womb or could not do so securely. These very early pregnancy losses often happen without the woman ever knowing she had conceived at all.

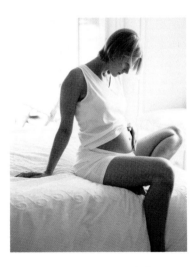

ABOVE By the time you reach this stage, the chances of miscarriage are tiny. However, whether you have had a previous miscarriage or whether this is the first time you have tried for a baby, both parents can increase their chances of a pregnancy which results in a healthy, full-term son or daughter using the Self-help and Preconceptual care suggestions on pages 34-74 before they conceive.

MISCARRIAGES
Only 1% of miscarriages happen after 12 weeks.

But the fact that it happens to so many couples does not make it any easier to cope with. Losing a pregnancy, even if it was not initially planned (which up to two-thirds are not) and even if it was at a very early stage, can feel like the cruellest and most devastating of blows.

Neither does it help that, for approximately half of all miscarriages, no one can even tell you why it happened. Many specialists explain it as being the body's own way of making sure it allows only healthy pregnancies to progress, as between 50 and 60% of the time pregnancy loss is associated with a chromosomal abnormality in the fetus or embryo. This may in part explain why miscarriage becomes progressively more common as women grow older. At 35-39 a woman has about a 20% risk; at 42+ this has risen to a risk of 40% or more.

Yet, if you have lost a baby in this way, there is a very good chance indeed (about 80%) that your next pregnancy will work out. Even if you have had three miscarriages one after the other, there is still a 60% chance that your next pregnancy will be fine.

However, for 1 in every 100 couples who has experienced one or more miscarriages, it will happen repeatedly. This is not the same as infertility, as they can clearly conceive, but the problem is sustaining the pregnancy. There is no single cause for recurrent miscarriages, but many different factors may play a part. These include:

BLOOD-CLOTTING DISORDERS

A woman's blood becomes thicker and stickier when she is pregnant. However, it becomes thicker in some women than in others. This may cause small blood clots to form in the blood vessels leading to and from the placenta. The clots may obstruct these important vessels that carry food and oxygen to the developing baby, and waste products away from him or her. There are certain substances that make your blood clot more easily, called antiphospholipid antibodies. New treatments to reduce the levels of these have been developed.

GENETICS

Although chromosomal problems are thought to be the cause of around 60% of miscarriages, they are usually random ones. Only 3–5% of couples who experience a miscarriage do so because they themselves have a chromosomal abnormality that is being passed to their unborn baby.

HORMONES

Probably the most common hormonal problem associated with recurrent miscarriage is too much luteinizing hormone. Around half all the women affected by polycystic ovary syndrome (see page 115) tend to make too much of it.

INFECTION

The possibility that infection may well play a role in later pregnancy loss is well accepted by most gynaecologists. The bugs responsible are thought to include toxoplasmosis, for instance, which may be found in cat faeces, raw meat and unpasteurized cheese. Yet although genital infections such as cytomegalovirus (which causes genital warts), mycoplasma and ureaplasma (see Bug-busting, page 40) and chlamydia have also been linked with miscarriage and difficulties in becoming pregnant in the first place, many specialists still feel it's unnecessary to check for these. However, this book's preconceptual care advisors strongly recommend a broad screening for all possible bugs that could affect fertility and pregnancy (see Bug-busting, page 40).

AN UNUSUALLY SHAPED WOMB

It is estimated that up to 10% of women who miscarry repeatedly have an unusually shaped womb. Yet many perfectly successful pregnancies have come from some very oddly shaped uteri, so there are no firm rules on this one.

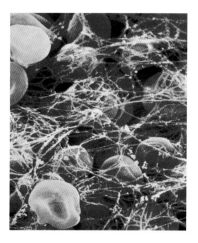

ABOVE This picture shows blood cells and proteins forming a tiny blood clot in a capillary. If your blood clots too easily, it can affect your pregnancy.

LIFESTYLE AND WORK

These factors can have a major effect on your chances of conceiving a healthy baby, and carrying him or her safely to term. The good news is that many are under your control, and so, wherever possible and practical, you could actively choose to change them for the better. See sections on:

- Your healthy home (page 67)
- At work (page 63)
- What's your poison? (page 38)
- Drugs and medicines (page 71)
- The fillings in your teeth (page 55)
- Fertility foods (page 50)
- Stress and infertility (page 59)
- Body weight matters (page 36)
- Emotional health (page 42)
- Which contraception? (page 44)

What Can Cause Fertility Problems in Men?

Around one-third of infertility problems are thought to be down to the male partner, and 30-40% related to both the man and the woman. Fortunately, fertility difficulties such as low sperm count can be rewardingly responsive to simple measures such as stopping smoking, taking nutritional supplements, clearing the system of harmful chemical residues (see the sections At work, page 63, and Your healthy home, page 67) and heavy metals (for example, mercury from fillings).

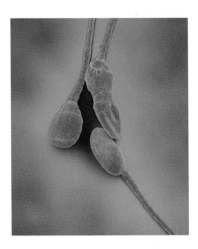

ABOVE It is normal for a proportion of the sperm cells in semen to be unusually formed: the one in the middle here, for instance, has a double head. But as long as around 30% or more are normal and relatively lively, there is a good chance of starting off a healthy pregnancy.

Semen analysis

The first thing a clinic would do for a man concerned about his fertility would be to analyse a sample of his semen. This needs to be ejaculated into a sterile plastic pot with a lid – the lab or your doctor would provide a container – and delivered to the laboratory as soon as possible, because up to three-quarters of your sperm will die in that sample jar within 3–6 hours of leaving your body. Many clinics have a quiet room to give men the privacy to produce a semen sample so it can be handed over right away.

The lab technicians will check the following:

- *How much semen has been ejaculated?* If only very little semen is produced, this may suggest a partial blockage in one or both vas deferens tubes which brings semen from the testicles to the penis tip. Scanty semen may suggest an infection in the testes or prostate. Some men are born with low sperm counts, or it could also be that the testes are simply not working very well.
- *Are any sperm present?* If the sample contains no sperm at all, this could be due to a wide variety of factors, including infection that has affected the parts of the body which produce sperm or caused a blockage in the tubes of the reproductive system. There is also the possibility of testicular failure.
- *How many sperm are in the semen?* Above 20 million per ml is felt to be OK; over 60 million per ml is looking good. Below 20 million per ml is felt to be too low. But numbers aren't everything. A man with a count of 10 million per ml whose sperm are mostly healthy and active has a similar chance of getting his partner pregnant as a man whose count is 100 million per ml but who has a high proportion, say 85% or more, of abnormal or stationary sperm.
- *How active are the sperm?* Sperm need to be swimming strongly and straight to be able to reach and fertilize an egg. A proportion of them will always be found to be going around in circles, stationary, shaking on the spot, weaving from side to side, or dead. They may

HOW MUCH IS ENOUGH?

An infection is a very common reason for not producing much ejaculate (say, just 1.5 ml or so). The average amount is 3-4 ml each time, but if you have not ejaculated for a couple of weeks, it would be nearer 10 ml. If you ejaculated the day before, it's likely to be nearer 0.5 ml, so let your doctor know when you last made love or masturbated if they are checking out your semen volume.

also be clumped together. The lab would grade them from 0 to 4 (0 means stationary, 3 is normal, and 4 positively turbo-charged). Pollutants from sources such as the surrounding air, home or work environment, tobacco and alcohol may all damage sperm.

- *What proportion are normally shaped?* Some sperm have double heads or short tails and so will find it more difficult to fertilize an egg properly because they may not be able to reach it or break inside. Some studies show abnormal sperm can often get into the Fallopian tubes all right, and that they do fertilize eggs, but that the resulting pregnancy is more likely to miscarry. Fertility experts usually feel that if semen contains 70% or more abnormal sperm this presents a significant problem.

If your semen analysis has found any problems, you will be offered further tests and investigations to find the cause. These additional tests are aimed at finding out some additional vital things about your sperm, such as the following:

- *Can they swim through your partner's cervical mucus and into her womb, then up her Fallopian tubes?* The main test to find this out is called a post-coital test (PCT). The fertility clinic lab needs to see a sample taken from your partner's cervix soon after you have had sexual intercourse with her. The sample will be a delicate mixture of her cervical mucus and your sperm cells. They can use this to check whether your sperm are able to swim through and reach the womb on the other side.

  If your sperm seem to be having trouble, the clinic would then check to see if your partner's body is making antibodies to your sperm and fighting them as if they were invading bacteria. This is not that unusual, and may sometimes explain why a woman can get pregnant with one man, but not with another.
- *Can your sperm break inside the waiting egg and fertilize it?* The laboratory could test for this with a 'hamster egg test' (which uses just that, with its outer barrier removed).

Other possibilities

RETROGRADE EJACULATION
Retrograde ejaculation (semen ejaculating backwards into your bladder) is a relatively rare condition. A urine test could check for it, since semen is a high-protein substance and produces bubbles when disturbed – like egg whites being beaten into a froth. Bubbles in the urine could indicate retrograde ejaculation.

HORMONAL PROBLEMS
Though hormonal treatments for a low sperm count are usually the first option people ask about, specialists estimate that only between 1 and 5% of men are infertile or subfertile because they are not making

WHY SPERM COUNT VARIES
Don't take a single sperm count as Gospel – their accuracy varies wildly. When the British Andrology Society sent samples from a single batch of semen to 20 different labs they got 20 different sperm count results. These varied from 1 million sperm per ml to 200 million per ml.

You may want to consider having two or three different tests over a period of a few weeks. A series of tests would also cater for the fact that your sperm count can vary over a few weeks anyway. Being tired, very stressed or upset, ill, not eating properly, smoking more than usual, having had a one-off drinking binge recently with the boys (see page 47), a sudden increase in exercise or even making love the night or morning before the test can all cause a temporary drop in sperm count.

Men's fertility also declines in the summer; several studies have found that sperm counts fall and that there is an increase in the number of malformed sperm during the warmer months.

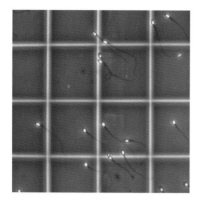

ABOVE This is a semen analysis test. The healthy sperm are the ones which have managed to reach the top section of the grid.

enough of any particular hormone. You can check on hormone levels with blood tests, and the one usually checked for is not testosterone, as most of us would have thought, but follicle-stimulating hormone (FSH) because it is the one which stimulates the formation of sperm cells.

GENETICS

Very occasionally there is a genetic reason for the complete absence of sperm. The most common of these is Klinefelter's syndrome in which, instead of the normal male XY chromosome, the man is born with an additional X chromosome, making him XXY. Usually a man with this syndrome does not make any sperm at all, and, since it is not treatable, the couple would be asked if they would like to consider trying donor insemination instead.

HEAT

Too much heat kills sperm. Testicles can become overheated if you sit for too long, wear tight trousers and underpants or work in a hot environment (see At work, page 63). Some doctors feel that varicose veins around the testicles called varicoceles could overheat the testes and reduce sperm count too (see page 48).

STRESS

Stress may be a factor (see Stress and infertility, page 59) since it can affect sperm count and hormone production. However, if you are under considerable stress and not fertile at the moment, this does not necessarily mean that there are no other physical factors as well.

RIGHT Jobs involving very long working days and a high stress quotient can affect men's fertility.

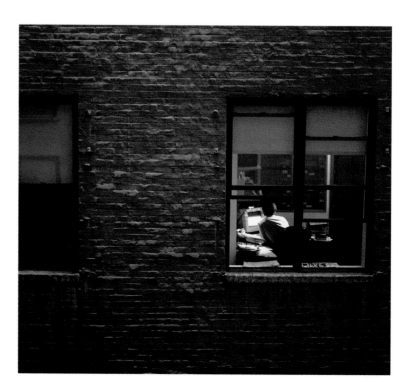

Medical Treatments – What's Available?

Three to four months in a good preconceptual care programme just may be the most helpful three months you ever spend. It can pay dividends by helping you make the most of the fertility you both have naturally. You may become pregnant without needing medical treatment. And, at the very least, if you and your partner are in the best possible physical and emotional shape after some preconceptual care this will maximize the chances of any of the medical or high-tech treatments working for you.

A short period of preconceptual care may be especially helpful for women who are in their late thirties and early forties, even though their natural fertility is declining faster than that of someone in their early thirties – unless their specialist gives a very good medical reason why they ought to start a medical treatment immediately rather than spend the next three to four months improving their health first.

Complementary health treatments

Complementary treatments often work well in conjunction with medical treatments, at a fraction of the cost. They can also form an important part of a preconceptual care programme to make the very most your fertility potential and improve general physical and mental health before starting any treatments. Conventional medicine does not have all the answers and neither do complementary therapies. Yet both have a great deal to offer, especially if they can work together.

There is extensive published clinical research which shows that several of the therapies – especially homeopathy, Chinese herbalism, Western herbalism and acupuncture – can be effective at combating certain fertility problems.

FIRST THINGS FIRST
Before paying out for expensive infertility treatments, spend at least three months (preferably four) getting yourself and your partner into the best physical and mental shape possible to enhance and maximize your own natural fertility.

The clinic jungle

Infertility is now big business in both Britain and America. If there is a growth industry in medicine, this is it. And very profitable it is too, as the cost of private medical care is not just keeping pace with inflation but growing inexorably by 10–15% every year.

If you badly want a baby but it's not happening, you can feel very vulnerable and find yourself spending a great deal of money to find out why, and to buy treatment. For instance, the average cost of just a single private IVF attempt is roughly $4,000 in America and £2,500 in the UK. Prices are comparable world-wide. Unfortunately, some clinics are more ethical – and honest with clients – than others. It is well worth while taking time and care in choosing one you feel happy with.

As a paying client at a private clinic, rather than a patient at a state-funded clinic, you theoretically have some control, and the valuable

SUCCESS RATES

Success quotients vary considerably. Clinics may say they achieve 'success' rates as high as 15–40%, which sounds pretty impressive when you think that in the general population only 10–15% of women trying to conceive naturally would become pregnant each month. But that's the pregnancy rate, not the number of people who have a live, healthy baby at the end of it. IVF pregnancies are in fact more likely to miscarry or be ectopic than natural pregnancies, and their 'take-home baby' rates are nearer 15–20%.

opportunity to find a clinic that suits you best and you feel most comfortable in. Some couples prefer a smaller, friendlier clinic where they can see the same doctors each time; others feel more confident at a big teaching hospital-based unit, headed by a famous obstetrician.

BE CLINIC-WISE
Try to do some homework first.

- Get hold of clinic league tables. In the UK the Human Fertilization and Embryology Authority (HFEA) is the licensing authority for infertility clinics and it produces league tables which show how successful they are. Check your country's equivalent.
- Read the leaflet *Choosing a Clinic* published by the organization called CHILD (see Helplines, page 139).
- Shop around. Ring up and ask for several clinic brochures.
- Pick perhaps three that you like the sound of, and which are geographically within reach. The latter is more important than it first sounds because repeatedly travelling far for tests and treatments can be a major additional source of stress when you have quite enough of it already.
- Visit those clinics if you can. Or ask to speak to a senior counsellor or their clinic director, and ask them as many questions as you can think of over the phone.

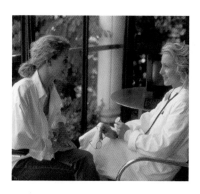

ABOVE If possible, try to meet the specialist who will be in charge of your treatment in person before you make the final choice of clinic. Do you feel comfortable with them, and do they inspire you with confidence without overselling what medical treatment could do for you? What does your partner think?

SOME QUESTIONS TO ASK WHEN CHOOSING A CLINIC

- Do the consultants have any special interest and expertise in any particular types of infertility (e.g. for women with blocked tubes, men with very low sperm count)?
- Do any of the consultants also work in the public infertility sector? If so, who and where?
- What treatments and tests do they offer?
- Do they have any restrictions as to who they take on (for example, due to age, former unsuccessful treatments)? Many have – because, for instance, if they accept women over 42 this will make their success rate look lower than, say, a clinic that only takes on younger couples.
- Have they got a waiting list?
- How successful are they with couples around the same age as yourselves with your type of difficulty if already diagnosed; for example, ovulation problems?
- Are there 'hidden' costs, like drugs, diagnostic tests, counselling and anaesthetic charges, and, if so, what are they?
- What is their take-home, or live birth rate?

Which Treatment?

If you decide to try assisted conception, consider beginning gently with lower-tech treatments first – so long as your doctors agree that they might be appropriate, and there is no good medical reason why you need to go straight to high-tech options. The latter are a last resort, not a first port of call. For instance, if you have unexplained infertility it might be helpful to begin with IUI (intra-uterine insemination), but if diagnostic tests have shown you have severely blocked tubes there would be no point and you would need to go straight for *in-vitro* fertilization (IVF).

Insemination techniques – helping nature along

These treatments involve placing a sample of sperm into the cervix (neck of the womb) or into the womb itself (IUI). The sample could be from your husband or male partner, or, if necessary, from a donor. Women having this type of treatment are sometimes also given fertility drugs, even if they are ovulating normally.

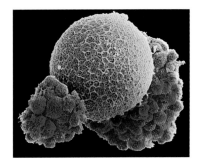

ABOVE This is a healthy human egg, which has recently been ovulated. The fluffy cells around it are called the cumulus corona cells. Their job is to nourish and protect the egg until it has been fertilized, and implanted itself in the womb.

Assisted insemination is suitable where there is some physical difficulty in getting the sperm to the right place. For example, it can be used for retrograde ejaculation, where sperm is fired backwards up into the bladder; or for men with potency problems because of a condition such as severe diabetes or MS. It is not helpful for a low sperm count or a high proportion of abnormal sperm unless donor semen is used.

DONOR INSEMINATION

If a male partner does not have enough normal, motile sperm to try for IVF or GIFT (see page 127), and treatments do not improve its quality or count, possible options include ICSI (see page 129) or considering a pregnancy achieved using donor sperm. The decision to go for this may be a complicated and difficult one for a couple, as it involves many issues both ethical, religious, personal and legal.

Donors are screened carefully. They may be medical students, husbands of other obstetric patients, college students or local businessmen. Clinics also take great care to match the characteristics of the male partner to a suitable donor, taking into account things like height, ethnic background, and hair and eye colour.

Most clinics will only treat married couples or those in long-term heterosexual relationships, but a few will also help lesbian couples.

Encouraging ovulation

This is usually the first treatment a clinic will try if they find that you are not ovulating (or doing so very erratically) despite the fact that both your Fallopian tubes and your partner's sperm are normal.

Most of the drugs used for this can have unpleasant side-effects, ranging from nausea and insomnia to fainting and mood swings. Complementary therapies which may help encourage healthy, regular ovulation include acupressure (see page 90), reflexology (see page 97), homeopathy (see page 78), herbalism (see page 82), Autogenic Training (see page 101), hypnotherapy (see page 100), relaxation and visualization techniques (see page 104).

The different types of conventional medication for helping women to ovulate include the following:

- *Clomiphene citrate*: This will encourage you to ovulate if you are not doing so naturally, and can also help if you have erratic or long cycles.
- *Bromocriptine*: This suppresses a hormone called prolactin, which you produce to make milk when breast-feeding, but also when you are under prolonged levels of stress. High amounts of prolactin in your bloodstream can stop ovulation; lower levels may still interfere with it.
- *Human chorionic gonadotrophin (HCG)*: This is the hormone that you make naturally when you are first pregnant. It makes an ovary release its 'dominant' follicle (that is the ripest) and also helps keep your womb lining in place, so it does not shed as usual in the form of a period.
- *Follicle-stimulating hormone (FSH)*: Your pituitary gland releases this from the first day of your period, and throughout the beginning of the rest of your menstrual cycle. Its job is to stimulate a group of follicles growing on the ovary's surface to ripen. FSH controls ovulation, in partnership with luteinizing hormone (LH). FSH may help women who have polycystic ovary syndrome to balance their high levels of LH.
- *Human menopausal gonadotrophin (hMG)*: This is, as its name suggests, made from the urine of women who have passed their menopause. A powerful drug, hMG may be used for women for whom clomiphene does not work. It contains both FSH and LH hormones. Monitoring of the drug's effect is essential, as there is a high risk of multiple births. It may help women who do not have periods.
- *Gonadotrophin-releasing hormone (GnRH)*: Normally made by the hypothalamus gland and released in pulses 90 minutes apart, the function of GnRH is to stimulate the release of LH and FSH. If a woman has lost a lot of weight over a short period of time, by dieting perhaps, or if she has anorexia, she will not release very much GnRH.
- *Gonadotrophin-releasing analogues*: Synthetic forms of GnRH are given in the form of an injection or nasal spray and thus give a constant rather than a pulsed dose. They may help women having IVF treatments, as they are thought to stimulate the production of more 'mature' eggs ready to be fertilized.

NO RHYME OR REASON
For one in five couples, doctors can find no reason for their infertility.

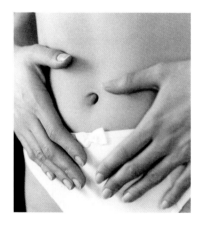

ABOVE The list of different drugs (see list right) can all help a woman to ovulate. When some women release an egg, either naturally or as a result of medication (often it's several, with ovulation drugs), they feel a pain or a dull ache on one side of their abdomen just where their ovaries are. It may be fleeting, or you may be aware of it on and off for up to 24 hours.

Clearing blocked tubes

A third of all women investigated for infertility have blocked or damaged Fallopian tubes, usually caused by an ongoing or past pelvic infection, endometriosis, previous abdominal surgery or a previous ectopic pregnancy. Depending on whereabouts along their length the trouble is, and the degree of damage to the lining of these delicate tubes, micro-surgery can sometimes solve the problem.

Pregnancy rates are 35–60% if adhesions that need to be removed from around the ovaries, and anything between 25 and 70% if there is a blockage *inside* the tubes which is treated with microsurgery.

Assisted conception techniques

GIFT (GAMETE INTRA-FALLOPIAN TRANSFER)

Although very popular in the 1980s to mid-1990s, GIFT is now no longer used very often. It involves mixing the couple's ripe eggs and sperm, then putting the mixture into one of the woman's Fallopian tubes so that fertilization can take place where it naturally would anyway. Pregnancy rates of 25–30% are quoted. Seen these days as a sophisticated method of artificial insemination, or a simplified form of IVF, it can only be used if the Fallopian tubes are healthy and not blocked. GIFT is suitable for couples for whom doctors can find no reason for their infertility or women with cervical mucus problems, because the technique bypasses the mucus barrier across the cervix. It is also worth trying if the woman is making antibodies to her partner's sperm (although sometimes these antibodies also exist in her womb and tubes).

GIFT-ET

This is a more recent technique, involving a combination of old-fashioned GIFT and IVF. Three of the woman's ripe eggs are collected by a hollow needle, guided by ultrasound. One or two are mixed with a sample of her partner's fresh semen, and the mixture is then put into one of her Fallopian tubes. At the same time, a single egg that has been fertilized in lab conditions is placed in her womb. Using both approaches together appears to be more successful than either used on their own.

IVF (IN-VITRO FERTILIZATION)

In this technique the woman's eggs are fertilized with her partner's sperm in a laboratory, and the resulting very young embryos (four to eight cells big) are placed back in the womb so they can implant in the lining there. Sometimes if several IVF attempts have failed, this is combined with 'assisted hatching', in which a tiny hole is made using a needle or chemical in the embryo's casing, so it can attach itself more easily to the womb lining.

IVF is suitable for women whose Fallopian tubes are damaged, who have endometriosis and sometimes for women who have 'unexplained' infertility (that is, where no reason can be found for it).

INCREASING YOUR CHANCES
Progressive obstetricians sometimes now suggest that women who are having IVF treatment may benefit from reflexology or herbal treatments just beforehand to increase their chances of conception.

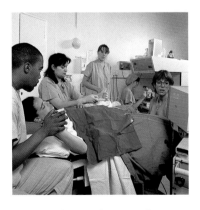

ABOVE With IVF and GIFT-ET, the woman's ripened eggs need to be collected via a minor operation, during which she remains awake though gently sedated, and often supported by her partner. The medical team uses a laparoscopic technique, involving a fine needle guided carefully by ultra-sound, to retrieve the eggs.

Improving semen quality

The main types of semen problem are low sperm count, a high proportion of damaged or abnormal sperm, sperm which are not moving normally, and either no sperm or none which are alive. Sometimes there may be a combination of two or more of these factors.

Before you request any medical treatment, there are many measures that a man can implement for himself first which may improve semen quality (see Preconceptual care for men, page 46). These improvements may be so great he no longer needs any clinical help. At the very least, they can make the very most of his own natural fertility potential, so that any treatments he does have are more likely to be successful.

So that you can tell whether these self-help measures make a difference, have a semen analysis (not just a straightforward number count) *before* you begin your preconceptual care programme. After four months of this, have another. Compare the results – your doctor or clinic can help you interpret them.

If there hasn't been enough – or indeed any – improvement, there are several useful medical treatment options available. These include:

- *Antibiotics*: These may be prescribed if there is an infection in the testes or seminal vesicles. This treatment is suitable for men whose sperm are abnormally shaped, or men producing only small amounts of ejaculate (though the volume does reduce anyway as they get older).
- *Cortisone*: This will reduce inflammation if a low-grade infection is suspected, or if there is evidence of sperm antibodies.
- *Sperm pre-selection*: This effectively skims off the best ones by spinning the sample with a cell culture medium in a medical centrifuge. These *crème de la crème* sperm can then be used for assisted fertilization techniques such as IUI, IVF, GIFT or ICSI.
- *Pentoxifylline*: If the sperm are normally formed but sluggish, this caffeine-like drug may also be added to their environment to make them livelier. This is suitable for men with low sperm counts or men whose sperm are not moving well.

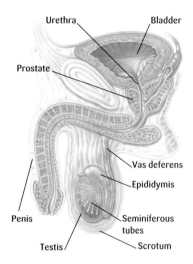

Urethra   Bladder
Prostate
Vas deferens
Epididymis
Penis
Seminiferous tubes
Testis
Scrotum

ABOVE A cross-section shows a man's reproductive and urinary system.

Treating male hormonal problems

As discussed earlier, although this is almost always the first treatment couples ask about, very few men are infertile because they are short of one particular hormone. Even when they are, the culprit is seldom testosterone, as most people would think.

Unfortunately, several clinics are still using hormonal drugs like clomiphene, testosterone and the anti-oestrogen tamoxifen to improve sperm count and quality, even though the research evidence suggests they are not that effective. HCG and hMG (see page 126) may be more help, and can be used either in combination or separately for men who are not making enough of the sperm-maturing LH and FSH.

Bromocriptine may be used if a man has high levels of the hormone prolactin, which can be caused by stress. In men, too much prolactin can produce loss of sex drive and impotence.

Dealing with blocked sperm-carrying tubes

Blockages are usually the result of an infection in the genito-urinary system. It may be a current one, or it may be an old one that healed long ago, leaving scarring or adhesions behind. These can partially or totally block one or more vital tubes. It does not take much to do so – the two vas deferens passages, for instance, whose job it is to take sperm from the epididymis to the urethra during ejaculation, are only the thickness of a fine guitar string inside.

Other possible blockage sites include the sperm-producing seminiferous tubes, which lie curled up like a ball of fine spaghetti in the testes; or the epididymis tubes which act as sperm reservoirs, storing it until it is ejaculated.

Microsurgery can be successful in clearing a blockage, but it depends where the problem is, and how much it is obstructing the tubes.

Helping retrograde ejaculation

If there is no sperm to be seen at all, it may be that the testes have been damaged in some way, or that the sperm is backfiring into the bladder when it is ejaculated. Drugs can be used to keep the bladder neck shut so the man can ejaculate and the sperm sample can be collected. It can then be used for a technique such as IUI, GIFT, IVF or ICSI.

When sperm cannot fertilize the egg

If this is the problem there are several different techniques that can be used to help the sperm break into the egg successfully. These include certain drugs which can enhance the acrosome reaction – the process where the bag of enzymes on the sperm's head bursts on contact with the egg, dissolving enough of its shell to let the sperm break inside. A caffeine wash is also used sometimes to give sperm added momentum. However, it is becoming increasingly common to use ICSI instead.

WHAT IS ICSI?
The substance the egg cell is made of is called cytoplasm, and ICSI (intra-cytoplasmic sperm injection) involves selecting one single healthy sperm (which does not even have to be moving) and inserting it directly through the cell's shell. This allows it to by-pass all the natural barriers – cervical mucus, eggshell and distance – that would usually confront it.

ICSI is also used for cases of 'unexplained infertility' where tests have found nothing wrong with sperm nor any problems on the woman's side. (One in five couples with unexplained infertility have a fertilization problem.) It is also suitable for men whose sperm count is very low or of poor quality, and for whom either DIY improvement techniques (see page 128) or medical treatments have not worked. ICSI can also help men who have difficulties getting an erection or ejaculating, for example those with severe diabetes, multiple sclerosis or spinal cord injury.

The treatment is also offered to couples for whom IVF has not worked, or to men who are making healthy sperm which cannot be ejaculated because of a blockage in the male reproductive plumbing system.

Pregnant? Hooray!

Just got the results of a positive pregnancy test? How do you feel - terrific or a little taken aback for no good reason that you can put your finger on?

Trying to conceive can send the emotional registers of the calmest couples on a white knuckle ride for months, even for years if it did not come easily. And ironically, getting the blue line or ring signal from a pregnancy test that says *yes, you've done it!* can do the same.

Reported reactions from women - and men - vary wildly from bursting into tears (variously attributed to delight, relief and pure shock), to simply not mentioning the subject for weeks and going on a spending spree that would make Ivana Trump blanche.

That's OK. It's allowed. Immediate happiness and total confidence when you find out you're pregnant is normal, but so are ambivalence and even downright alarm. Don't let those advertisements for pregnancy kits showing ecstatic couples hugging, or the expectations of others tell you any different. Your reactions are your own, they are as individual and unique as you are, and you are entitled to them. They may be a result of difficulties you have had becoming pregnant, past pregnancies, your own childhood, issues surrounding your relationship with your partner, work, home or your financial situation.

Yet you have got nine months to get comfortable with the idea, with its implications and to work through anything that you may not yet be sure about or that is not yet as you need it to be. As one elderly and internationally respected psychologist from Santa Barbara put it: 'It can be a shock to get what you've always wanted. But hey - it gets better.'

How much better? If what other new parents say is true, better than any non-parent ever thought possible.

Pregnant? Hooray!

When it's happened for you

Never mind how many pregnancies occur each year. If it's happened to you and you want it, it feels like a miracle. An ordinary miracle maybe, one that happens to thousands of couples every day, but a miracle nonetheless – especially if you have had some difficulties conceiving, or it has taken you longer than you thought.

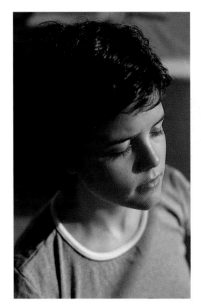

ABOVE International research suggests that both spoken and unspoken (psychic) communication between mother and unborn baby can begin very early on – some believe as early as the first few days after conception. What's more, if you or your partner talk out aloud to your unborn child, Irish pre-natal research suggests your baby can hear, probably through sound-vibration receptors in their tiny skeleton, as early as 17 weeks, even though their actual ears do not form until 33 weeks.

If this has been the case for you and your partner, becoming pregnant at last is a terrific achievement and one to be very proud of indeed. If you conceived easily and naturally, it's also a cause for major congratulations and rejoicing – especially if you have been taking all that trouble to follow a preconceptual care programme and implement some of the suggestions outlined in this book. They'll have all taken time, careful thought and discipline, but both you and your tiny embryo are reaping the benefits already.

You: if you have been following your own preconceptual care system for the last few months, you and your partner are probably feeling healthier and better than you have felt for many years, besides having achieved a much-wanted pregnancy. *Your baby?* The benefits start early. Very early. Day One and before, as a matter of fact.

We think babies in the womb are insulated in a protective cocoon, shielded from the toxins and shocks of the outside world. And we imagine that they will get all the nourishment needed from their mother, no matter how she is doing. That time in the womb is a free period, with few consequences for anything a mother does, or is exposed to. But that is true only up to a point.

For good or ill, a fetus the size of a pinhead is already developing the equipment (both emotional and physical) that will serve them for a lifetime. Their spine is forming at three weeks, their heart at five. They make their first movements at six. That's how fast it all happens.

Increasingly, research is showing that what happens to an expectant mother – what she eats, what she breathes, the good and bad experiences she has – can affect her unborn baby right from the date of fertilization when it is too small to see with the naked eye, for the rest of

VISUALIZING YOUR BABY
If you are pregnant, take a few minutes each day to close your eyes, breathe deeply, and see in you mind's eye your future baby burrowing safely into your womb lining and staying there, growing, safe and secure. Send thought-messages of love and welcome to him or her, telling them they are wanted and safe.

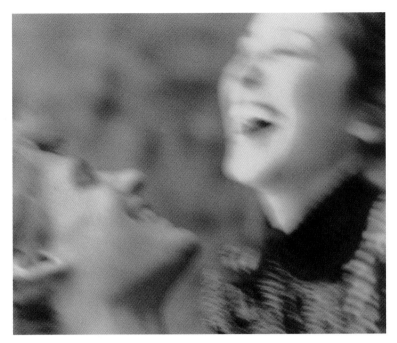

LEFT Some couples find they want to share their happiness and excitement as soon as they conceive. For others, especially if conception took a while to happen, this remains a quiet and private time of delight, and hope, for much longer – often until the pregnancy begins to be obvious, from around four or five months.

his or her life. One important example from the nutrition point of view is the medical advice for women to take folic acid supplements before they even try to conceive, because a higher rate of spina bifida has been documented in babies born to women who were short of folic acid when they became pregnant.

From the life experiences point of view, there is a wealth of international research from America, Ireland, Spain, Venezuela, France, Australia and Britain suggesting that babies are aware of their mothers' emotions in the womb and that a relatively calm pregnancy tends to produce calmer babies, and that a stressful life during pregnancy can affect a baby's neurological circuitry for good. That can have many different potential effects ranging from left-handedness to impaired ability to deal with stress when they grow up (see References, page 136).

Babies born to women who have not been eating properly are born lighter than they should be (low birthweight). Groundbreaking research by Professor David Barker of Southampton University shows that what your baby weighs at birth can have a big impact on their health as they grow up. If a baby is too light or small at birth, he or she has a bigger risk of high blood pressure, heart disease and non-insulin-dependent diabetes. They are also more likely to develop asthma.

Avoiding miscarriage

However, the reverse is true for babies of normal weight, who are *less* likely to develop these disorders when they grow up. Research from Surrey University also suggests that if their mothers and fathers are properly nourished and have rid their bodies of environmental toxins before they conceive the resulting baby is a good deal less likely to

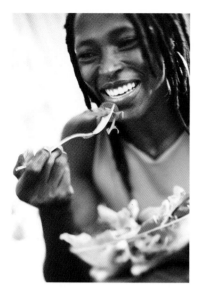

ABOVE If you have been able to follow a healthy diet containing plenty of fresh and raw fruit and vegetables while you were trying to conceive, good for you. Keep it going now you are pregnant!

miscarry as well. So, if you and your partner have been using a preconceptual care programme, you have already improved your chances of avoiding miscarriage, and having a baby who will be healthy when grown up.

This is very important. For one thing, many couples who have had difficulty becoming pregnant, or diagnosed fertility problems, find that, like couples who have experienced miscarriages, their trust that 'all will go well – why shouldn't it?' has gone. Their bodies didn't work as they were supposed to last time around and more than an echo of the insecurity, and the worry and guilt that can produce, may remain.

For another, it is also unfortunately true that there does seem to be a higher than average miscarriage rate for mothers who had difficulty conceiving, and also for women who have become pregnant as a result of assisted fertility treatments like IVF.

Early miscarriage is far more common than anyone usually realizes anyway. One study in 1996 looked at 200 women who were planning to become pregnant and had no history of fertility problems at all. The researchers found a 31% rate of early pregnancy loss. However, once you get past week 12, other research shows that the pregnancy loss rate plummets to just 1%, and continues to fall still further as your pregnancy progresses.

The uneasiness and ambivalence about an IVF pregnancy – or with finally being pregnant after a long struggle – can be compounded by the way that medical staff treat you. Your pregnancy may be labelled 'high risk'. You may well be urged to have a caesarean or induction too, because this is a precious baby who did not come easily. And, while additional care may be very welcome, it can also lead to extra monitoring, invasive testing and interventions which are (a) not always necessary and (b) serve to further medicalize the whole process, continually reminding you that something could go wrong.

However, there is still an enormous amount you can do to help ensure that your pregnancy brings you a healthy baby and an easier labour nine months from now. If you have been dipping into this book, you have probably come across most of it – but here is a summary for you anyway:

SEVEN STEPS FOR A POSITIVE PREGNANCY

1 Carry on eating healthily.
2 Avoid alcohol, cigarettes and all drugs unless they are medically necessary.
3 Cut down on stress in all areas of your life. Make room for your pregnancy – slow down. Don't try to power on as before.
4 Take time to consciously relax for a minimum of 10–15 minutes every single day. As you do, visualize your baby safe and secure in your womb.
5 Exercise regularly and gently (check with your doctor if not sure about type of exercise).

6 If you were supported by a complementary therapist while you were trying to become pregnant, stay in touch. They may be able to offer you continued treatments to help you stay well during pregnancy, have a smoother, calmer labour and give birth to a healthy baby.

7 If you have been taking nutritional supplements, check with a nutritionist right away that it is OK to carry on. If you have been taking herbal supplements, discontinue as soon as you have conceived, until you have checked with a qualified herbalist.

Good luck! Here's to your child of the future. May he or she be healthy and happy, and bring you great joy ...

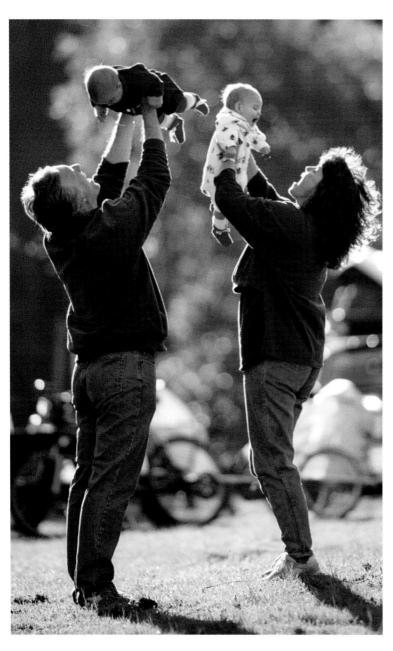

LEFT Remember that study by Surrey University on more than 367 couples mentioned earlier? The one where nearly 4 out of 10 of them had a history of infertility and repeated miscarriage – yet after a preconceptual care programme like the one outlined in this book, 9 out of 10 of them had their own babies?

None of those babies were born too early (before 36 weeks), none weighed less than 2.5 kg (5 lb 2 oz), none needed to go into a special babycare unit after birth, and there wasn't one single miscarriage or birth malformation amongst them. Those couples all had healthy, normal babies – like these two on the left.

If it worked for them, it could work for you, too.

References

SEASONS AND FERTILITY
'Differences in the quality of semen in outdoor workers during summer and winter', RJ Levine (1990) *N Engl J Med* 323.

HOW FIT AND WELL ARE YOU RIGHT NOW?
Chlamydia:
'Screening for chlamydia infections in women attending family planning clinics', J Schater *et al.* (1983) *West J Med* 138.
Overweight:
'Obesity: a never-ending cycle?', J Foreyt and WS Poston (1998) *Int J Fertil Women's Med* 43(2).
'Weight loss results in significant improvement in pregnancy and ovulatory rates in anovulatory obese women', AM Clark *et al.* (1995) *Hum Reprod* 10.
Smoking:
'Placental element levels in relation to foetal development of obstetrically normal births: a study of 37 elements', N Ward *et al.* (1987) *Int J Biosocial Res* 9(1).
Adverse effects on fertility:
Smoking & Reproduction, research studies factsheet, ASH (2000).
'Smoking and infertility', JM Campbell *et al.* (1979) *Med J Aust* 1.
'Relation between smoking and age of natural menopause', H Jick *et al.* (1977) *Lancet* 1.
Bug-busting:
Herpes: The ABC of Sexually Transmitted Diseases, MW Alder (1984) British Medical Assocation.
'The role of viruses in congenital defects', RJ Blattner (1974) *Am J Dis Child* 128.
Mycoplasmas:
'Mycoplasma infections and infertility', H Gnarpe, in Mancini (ed.) (1972) *Male Fertility & Sterility*, p. 114.
'Ureaplasmal infections of the male urinogenital tract, in particular prostatitis and semen quality', W Weidner (1982) *Urol Int* 40.

DRUGS
General Household Survey, Office of National Statistics (1997).
'Sex and drugs', in Nikki Bradford (1995) *Men's Health Matters*, Vermilion, pp. 373-376.
Benzodiazepines:
'... x24 increase in perinatal death' (1992) *Acta Obstet Gynecol Scand* 71.
Neurobehaviorial Teratology, B Yanai (ed.) (1984) Elsevier.
The Initial Investigation and Management of the Infertile Couple, Evidence Based Clinical Guidelines No 2, Royal College of Obstetricians and Gynaecologists (February 1998).
Drug abuse and alcoholism:
'Low serotonin levels due to tranquilliser damage' (1977) *Am J Psychiatry* 134: 665-669.
'Number of women given BZD in pregnancy' (1989) *Psychosomatics* 30: 25-31.
Youth at High Risk of Substance Abuse, KL Kumpfer, in BS Brown and AR Mills (eds) DHHS Publication no. 9, ADM, pp. 87-1537.
Tranx destroying fetal benzo receptors and thus their self calming mechanisms: (1986) *Neurobehav Toxicol Teratol* 8: 433-440.
'Drugs to avoid in pregnancy', A Shehata and C Nelson-Piercy (2000) *Curr Opin Obstet Gynecol* 10: 44-52.
'Chromosome breakages in users of marijuana', MA Stenchever *et al.* (1993) *Am J Obstet Gynecol* 53(3).
'Teratogenicity of cocaine in humans', N Bongol (1987) *J Pediatr* 1.
Paracetamol:
'Mutagenicity studies on paracetamol in human volunteers', J Kocisova *et al.* (1988) *Mutation Res* 209.
Painkillers and miscarriage:
'Environmental determinants of birth defects prevalence', G Watanabe (1979) *Contributions to Epidemiology and Biostatistics.*

AT WORK
Occupational Reproductive Hazards, Maureen Paul (1997) *Lancet* May 10.
See also medical databases REPROTOX (tel +1 202 293 5137) or the Teratogen Information System TERIS (tel +1 206 543 2465).
Chemicals and other work-related agents:
London Hazards Centre Factsheets: *Workplace Chemicals & Reproductive Health* (1993), sheet no. 40, *Physical Agents & Reproductive Health* (1993), sheet no. 41, *Women Hurt at Work* (1999), sheet No. 67.
'Reproductive health at work, part 1' (1998) *Hazards* 83.
'Reproductive health at work, part 2' (1998) *Hazards* 64.
Reproductive Hazards in the Workplace, LM Farzier (1997) Van Nostrand Reinhold.
Generations At Risk, How environmental toxins may affect reproductive health in Massachusetts (July 1996) (For details of report, tel +1 617 497 7440).
The Effects of Workplace Hazards on Male Reproductive Health, DHHS (NIOSH), NIOSH Publications Dissemination, 4676 Columbia Parkway, Cincinnati, OH, USA.
Protecting the Future, TUC report on health and safety for pregnant women (1998) TUC Publications, Congress House, Great Russell Street, London WC1B 3LS, UK.
One-Eyes Science: Occupational Health and Women Workers, Karen Messing (1998) Temple University Press.
VDU Terminal Sickness, Peggy Bentham (1994) Greenprint (currently out of print, but very helpful: ask if your library can find a copy).
'Effect of prolonged autovehicle driving on male reproductive function: a study among taxi drivers', Figa-Talamanca *et al.* (1996) *Am J Indust Med* 30.
'Male infertility and occupational exposures', Figa-Talamanca (1992) *J Occup Med Toxicol* 1.
'Fertility of male workers exposed to cadmium, lead or manganese', JP Gennart (1992) *Am J Epidemiol* 135.
'Fertility and semen quality of workers exposed to high temperatures in the ceramics industry', Figa-Talamanca and DellOrco (1992) *Reprod Toxicol* 6.
'Effects of workplace on fertility and related reproductive outcomes', B Baranksi (1993) *Environ Health Perspect* 101.
'Prospective assessment of fecundability of female semi-conductor workers', Eskenazi *et al.* (1995) *Am J Med* 28.
Male Mediated Developmental Toxicity, AF Olshan (1994) Plenum Press.
Ionizing and Non ionizing Radiations, R Brent *et al.* (1993) Williams and Wilkins.
'Reproductive effects of chemical exposures in health professions', G Ahlborg, Jnr (1995) *J Occup Environ Med* 37.
'Analysis of reproductive health hazard information on material safety data sheets for lead and ethylene glycol ethers', ME Paul (1994) *Am J Indust Med* 25.
Carpet Green Tag scheme, Anderson Laboratories Report (August 1992).

YOUR HEALTHY HOME
(1987) *Environ Res* 43: 290-307.
BRE Report No. 299, Construction Research Corporation Ltd (1996).
Prescriptions for a Healthy House, Paula Baker (1998) Inword Press.
'Benzene/cancer in painters and decorators' (1998) *Cancer Detect Prev* 22: 533-539.
'Unexplained infertility in women with high levels of decorating/furnishing chemicals: prolonged exposure to wood preservatives causes endocrine and immunological disorders in women', I Gerhard *et al.* (1991) *Am J Obstet Gynecol* 165(2).

'Your healthy house', *What Doctors Don't Tell You* (April 1999), vol 10, no 1.

STRESS

'Effect of psychological stress on human semen quality', Laura Fenster *et al.* (1997) *J Androl* March/April.

'Stress related reproductive failure', ER Barnea *et al.* (1991) *J IVF Embryo Transfer* 8.

'Somatic correlations with the unconscious repudiation of femininity in women', K Menninger (1939) *J Nerv Mental Dis* 89.

'Stress and semen quality in an in vitro fertilisation programme', KL Harrison *et al.* (1987) *Fertil Steril* 48.

'Performance anxiety in infertility treatment: effect on semen quality', KR Hammond *et al.* (1990) *Fertil Steril* 53.

'Effect of stress and characteristic adaptabilty on semen quality in healthy men', PT Giblin *et al.* (1988) *Fertil Steril* 49.

'Drug use and reproduction', RJ Stillman *Fertil Steril* (1985) 46.

'Spontaneous pregnancy in couples waiting for artificial insemination because of severe male infertility', R Mattoras *et al.* (1996) *Eur J Obstet Gynecol.*

'Spontaneous cure of male infertility', RH Glass and RJ Ericsson (1979) *Fertil Steril* 3.

'Treatment-independent pregnancy among infertile couples', JA Collins and W Wrixon (1983) *N Engl J Med* 309.

'Non therapy related pregnancies in the consorts of a group of men with obstructive azoospermia', AM Jequier (1985) *Andrologicia* 17.

HIS HEALTH

'Evidence for decreasing quality of semen in last 50 years', Carlsen *et al.* (1992) *BMJ* 305.

'Male fertility and occupation exposures', Figa-Talamanca (1992) *J Occup Med Toxicol* 1.

'Male reproductive health and environmental oestrogens', Editorial (1995) *Lancet* 345.

'Testosterone in chronic alcoholic men', M Irwin (1988) *Br J Addiction* 83.

'Effect of zinc administration on plasma testosterone, dihydrotestosterone and sperm count', (1981) *Arch Androl* 7.

'Selenium supplementation in sub fertile human males', R Scott *et al.* (1997) *Trace Elements in Man and Animals* 9, NRC Research Press, Ottawa.

'Growing up too soon', N Boyce (1997) *New Scientist* August 2.

'The human testes: an organ at risk?', Giwercman and N Skakkebaek (1992) *Int J Androl* 15.

Men's Health Matters, Nikki Bradford (1995) Vermilion.

FERTILITY FOODS

The Composition of Foods, MAFF/The Society of Chemistry (1991).

'Zinc and human male infertility', J Piesse (1983) *Int Clin Nutr Rev* 3.

'Effects of zinc deficiency on human reproduction', S Jameson (1976) *Acta Med Scand* 197A, Suppl 539.

'Adverse effects of zinc deficiency', (1995) *J Orthomol Med* 10(3 and 4) (republished by Foresight).

'Adverse effects of manganese deficiency on reproductive health', Tuula E Tuormaa (1996) *J Orthomol Med* 11(2): 69-79 (republished by Foresight).

'B6: the effects of pyridoxine on pituitary hormone secretion in amenorrhea-galactorrhea syndromes', GS Kidd *et al.* (1982) *J Clin Endocrinol Metab* 54(4).

Report, GE Abraham and JT Hargrove (1979) *World Med News*, March 19.

'Vit E: the effect of anti oxidant treatment on human spermatozoa and fertilisation rate in an in vitro fertilisation program', E Geva (1996) *Fertil Steril* 66(3).

'Treatment of infertility with vitamin E', R Bayer (1960) *Int J Infertil* 5.

'Vit C: Ascorbic acid protects against endogenous oxidative DNA damage in human sperm', CG Fraga *et al.* (1991) *Proc Natl Acad Sci USA* 88.

'Effects of ascorbic acid on male fertility', EB Dawson *et al.* (1987) *Ann NY Acad Sci* 498.

'Augmentative effects of ascorbic acid upon induction of human ovulation in clomiphene ineffective, anovulatory women', (1977) *Int J Fertil* 22(3).

WHEN PREGNANCY JUST ISN'T HAPPENING

'Abnormal sperm getting to Fallopian tubes: sperm transport and survival in women with special reference to the Fallopian tube', M Ahlegren *et al.* (1975) in *The Biology of Spermatazoa*, INSERM International Symposium, Basel.

'Abnormal sperm and miscarriage: endocrine patterns in term pregnancies following abortion', GES Jones *et al.* (1951) *J Am Med Assoc.*

COMPLEMENTARY THERAPIES

Herbs:

'Agnus Castus extracts inhibit prolactin secretion of rat pituitary cells', Sliutz *et al.* (1993) *Hormone Metab Res* 25.

'Treatment of corpus luteum insufficiency', D Propping and T Katzorke (1987) *Z Allgemeinmed* 63.

A Modern Herbal, Mrs M Grieve (1931) Penguin.

The Hamlyn Encyclopaedia of Complementrary Health, Nikki Bradford (ed.) (1996, 2000) Hamlyn.

The Complete Woman's Herbal, Anne McIntyre (1994, 1999) Gaia.

The Herb Users Guide, David Hoffman (1987) Thorsons.

Natural Healing in Gynaecology, R Nissim (1986) Pandora Press.

The British Herbal Phamacopoeia, British Herbal Medical Association.

Potters New Encyclopaedia of Botanical Drugs, Health Science Press.

Reflexology:

Reflexology: a Practical Approach, Vicki Pitman and Kay MacKenzie (1997) Stanley Thornes.

Reflexology & Unexplained Infertility, Helen Pearce (2000) The Association of Reflexologists.

'Has reflexology an effect on fertility?', Leila Eriksen (1994) Chairman of the Forenede Danske Zoneterapeuter (Danish Reflexology Association) Research Committee.

'Reflexology and infertility', Jane Holt (2000) *Reflextions*, March.

'How reflexology helped me conceive – a case study'. Melanie Bixby (1999) *Reflextions*, March.

Bach Flower Remedies:

The Illustrated Handbook of Bach Flower Remedies, Philip M Chancellor (2000) CW Daniel.

The Medical Discoveries of Edward Bach, Physician, Nora Weeks (1940) CW Daniel.

Bach Flower Remedies for Women, Judy Howard. CW Daniel.

Chinese herbal medicine/acupuncture/acupressure:

'Auricular acupuncture in the treatment of female infertility', I Gerhard and F Postneek (1992) *Gynaecol Endocrinol* September 6.

'The treatment of immunological infertility with Chinese medical herbs of ziyin jianghuo' (1995) *Chung-Kuo Chung His I Chieh Ho Tsa Chih* 15.

'Clinical and experimental study or composite wuzi dihuang liquor in treating male infertility', X-F Yang, T Wci and J Tong (1995) *Chung-Kuo Chung Hsi i Chieh Ho Tsa Chih* 15.

'Clinical Study on treatment of male infertility with shengjing pill', RA Chen and H Weh (1995) *Chung-Kuo Chung Hsi Chieh Ho Tsa Chih* 15(4).

'Effect on Nei-Yi recipe on plasma beta endorphin levels during menstrual cycle in women with endometriosis', CQ Yu *et al.* (1995) *Chung-Kuo Chung Hsi Chieh Ho Tsa Chih* 15(1).

Acupressure Step by Step: The Oriental Way to Health, Jacqueline Young (1994, 2001) Thorsons.

Aromatherapy:

(Bronchitis) JP Ferley and N Poutignat (1989) *Phytother Res* 3(3).

(Thrush) (1985) *Phytotherapy* 15, September.

Complementary Therapies in Medicine, CJ Stevenson (1994) Middlesex Hospital Intensive Care Unit.

Aromatherapy – A Nurse's Guide for Women, Ann Percival (1996) Amberwood.

Potters New Encyclopaedia of Botanical Drugs and Preparations, RC Wren. CW Daniel.

The Fragrant Pharmacy, V Wormwood (1991) Bantam.

The Directory of Essential Oils, Wanda Sellar (1992) CW Daniel.

'Aromatherapy and stress related symptoms', M Sprake *The Aromatherapist* 4(3).

'Aromatherapy and stress related health disorders', Hazel Charlesworth *The Aromatherapist* 2(4).

Hypnotherapy:

'Psychomatic sterility and psychosomatic infertility', A Chigbugh (1975) *Riv-Int Psicol Ipnosi* Jan–March 16(1): 37–41.

'Infertility and pregnancy loss – hypnotic interventions for reproductive challenges', in Horbyak *et al.* (eds) (2000) *The Use of Hypnosis in Women's Health Care*, The American Psychological Association, Washington DC.

'Simple hypnotherapy for infertility', in D Waxman (1989) *Hypnosis, the Fourth European Congress at Oxford*.

'Further gynaecological conditions treated by hypnotherapy', FH Leckie (1965) *Int J Clin Exp Hypnosis* 13: 11–25.

PREGNANT? HOORAY!

'Estimated rates of human fertility and pregnancy loss', M Zinaman and E Clegg (1996) *Fertil Steril* March 65(3).

The Miraculous World of Your Unborn Baby, Nikki Bradford (2001) Salamander Books.

'Weight in infancy and death from coronary heart disease', DJP Barker (1989) *Lancet* 11.

'Fetal and placental size and risk of hypertension in adult life', DJP Barker (1990) *BMJ* 301.

'Foetal and infant growth and impaired glucose tolerance at age 64', CN Hales *et al.* (1991) *BMJ* 303.

'The importance of nutrition around conception in the prevention of handicap', M Wynn and A Wynn (1981) *Appl Nutr I*, British Dietetic Association.

Editorial Consultants

Helplines

United Kingdom

The British Society for Mercury Free Dentistry: 221–223 Old Brompton Road, London SW5 0EA Tel. 020 7373 3655

CHILD: *support, information, resources and clinic information, for people experiencing fertility problems:* Charter House, 43 St Leonards Road, Bexhill-on-Sea, East Sussex TN40 1JA Tel. 01424 732361

FORESIGHT: *a wealth of expert advice and information on preconceptual care:* 28 The Paddock, Godalming, Surrey GU7 1XD Tel. 01483 427839

The Healthy House: *natural paints, water filters and hired EM radiation detection meters:* Cold Harbour, Ruscombe, Stroud, Gloucestershire GL6 6DA Tel. 01435 752216

The Human Fertilization and Embryology Authority: *government body who provide information on fertility clinic lists and league tables:* Paxton House, 30 Artillery Lane, London E1 7LS Tel. 020 7377 5077

ISSUE: The National Fertility Association: *advice and information on all aspects of infertility:* 114 Lichfield Street, Walsall WS1 1SZ Tel. 01922 722888

The London Hazards Centre: *advice, information and major resources on potential work health hazards and what to do about them:* Hampstead Town Hall Centre, 213 Haverstock Hill, London NW3 4QP Tel. 020 7794 5999

Marriage Care: *advice, information and training in natural family planning and fertility recognition:* Clitherow House, 1 Blythe Mews, Blythe Road, London W14 0NW Tel. 020 7371 1341

The Miscarriage Association: *support and information:* c/o Clayton Hospital, Northgate, Wakefield, West Yorkshire WF1 3JS Tel. 01942 200799

National Endometriosis Society: 50 Westminster Palace Gardens, Artillery Row, London SW1P 1RL Tel. 020 7222 2776

Patients Against Mercury Amalgam (PAMA): *information about mercury fillings and their safe removal as well as information on tests and treatments:* Mrs Kilmartin, Flat 9, 6–9 Bridgewater Square, London EC2Y 8AH Tel. 020 7256 2994

Quitline: *support and information for giving up smoking:* Freephone 0800 002200

The Soil Association: *campaigns for and information on organic food:* Bristol House, 40–56 Victoria Street, Bristol BS1 6BY Tel. 0117 929 0661

COMPLEMENTARY THERAPIES AND FINDING A PROFESSIONALLY QUALIFIED THERAPIST:

Acupuncture and Acupressure: The British Acupuncture Council Tel. 020 8735 0400

Aromatherapy: The Aromatherapy Organisations Council Tel. 020 8251 7912

Bach Flower Remedies: The Dr Edward Bach Centre Tel. 01491 834678

Chinese Herbal Medicine: The Register of Chinese Herbal Medicine Tel. 020 7470 8740

Homeopathy: The Society of Homeopaths Tel. 0870 7703214

Hypnotherapy: The National Register of Hypnotherapists and Psychotherapists Tel. 01282 716839

Meditation/visualization/relaxation: Friends of the Western Buddhist Order Tel. 020 8981 1225. Transcendental Meditation (TM): TM UK Tel. 08705 143733. Yoga: British Wheel of Yoga Tel. 01529 306851

Nutritionists: British Association of Nutritional Therapists Tel. 0870 6061284

Reflexology: The Association of Reflexologists Tel. 0870 5673320

Shiatsu: The Shiatsu Society Tel. 01788 555051

Western Medical Herbalists: National Institute of Medical Herbalists Tel. 01392 426022

If you cannot find a good practitioner in your area through the above organizations, or need advice about other complementary therapies, contact the Institute for Complementary Medicine Tel. 020 7237 5165

USA

The Dental Amalgam Mercury Syndrome Support Group (DAMS): P.O. Box 19032, Lakewood, CO 80226 Tel: (303) 238 1673

The March of Dimes: 1275 Mamaroneck Avenue, White Plains, NY 10605 Tel. (914) 428 7100

National Clearing House for Drug and Alcohol Information: 11426 Rockville Pike, Rockville, MD 20852 Tel. (800) 729 6686

National Center for Complementary and Alternative Medicine at the National Institutes of Health USA: NCCAM Clearinghouse, P.O. Box 7923, Gaithersburg, Maryland 20898 Tel. (866) 644 6226

National Institute of Environmental Health Issues: The Public Affairs Office, Research Triangle Park, NC 27709 Tel. (919) 541 3345

Parentcare: *for couples experiencing higher risk pregnancy/birth:* 9041 Colgate Street, Indianapolis, IN 46268 Tel. (317) 872 9913

Resolve: 1310 Broadway, Somerville, MA 02144, USA Tel. (617) 623 1156 Website: www.resolve.org

Australia

The Australian Council of Family Planning Inc: 36 Ferguson Street, P.O. Box 529, Forrestville, NSW 2087 Tel. (02) 9452 5244

Endometriosis Association of Victoria: 37 Andrew Crescent, South Croydon, Victoria 3136 Tel. (03) 9870 0536

The Fertility Society of Australia: Waldron Smith Management, 61 Danks Street, Port Melbourne, Victoria 3207 Tel. (03) 9645 6359

Natural Family Planning Sydney: Level 2, 276 Pitt Street, Sydney Tel. (02) 9390 5156

Index

A

abnormalities, babies with older
    mothers 13-14
achondroplasia 16
acrosome 20
acupressure 90, 92-3
acupuncture 90-1
age 12-16
agrimony 88
alcohol
    men 47
    women 39
alcohols, aromatherapy 94
aldehydes 94
allergies 37
alphafetoprotein (AFP) test 14
amenorrhoea 80
amniocentesis test 13, 14
amphetamines 75
anaerobic bacteria 49
anaesthetics 63
andropause 14-15
Angelica sinensis 83
anise-star, aromatherapy 95
Anthemis nobilis 85
anti-inflammatory drugs 72
antibiotics 72
    semen quality and 128
anticonvulsants 72
antifungal drugs 72
aromatherapy 94-6
ashwagandha 84, 85
assisted insemination 125
auricular therapy 97
autogenic training (AT) 101-2, 104, 105,
    107
Avena sativa 85
ayurvedic medicine 83-4

B

B vitamins 51
baby's sex, choosing 28, 29-31
Bach flower remedies 86-9
barrier contraceptives 45
benzene 67-8
benzodiazepines (BZDs) 73-4
bergamot oil 96
beta-blockers 72
birth defects, older mothers 13-14
blastocysts 21
blood loss, ovulation 24
blood test 36
blood-clotting disorders 119
body temperature 11
body weight

men 46-7
    preconceptual 36-7
boys, ways of choosing 28, 29-31
bromocriptine 126

C

cabbage 54
caffeine 54
candida 37
Candida 49
cannabis 75
carbon disulphide 63
carpets
    VOCs 69
cervical canal, 23
cervical mucus 11, 23, 24
    problems 117-18
cervical smear 36
cervix 23-4
    softening of 24
Chamaelirium luteum 83
chamomile 85
charting temperature 24-5
chase tree 83
chemicals
    at work 63-4
    pollution in the home 67-9
Chinese angelica 83
Chinese therapies 90-3
chlamydia 3, 40, 49
cholesterol 15
chorionic villi 21
chromosomes 29
cigarettes
    men 47-8
    women 38-9
clematis 87
climaxes 28
clinics 123-5
    choosing 124
    costs 123
clomiphene citrate 126
CMV 41
cocaine 75
coffee 54
combined pill 44
complementary therapies 7, 77-111
    and conventional treatments 123
computer screens 64-5
conception 17-20
condoms 45
congenital cataracts 15
contraception 44-5
contraceptive injections 45
cortisone, semen quality 128

coumarins 94
Cowper's gland 18
crack cocaine 75
cystic fibrosis 16
cystitis 27
cytomegalovirus (CMV) 41, 49

D

dairy products 54
damiana 84
Dang Gui 83
decorating, house 68-9
detoxing food 53-4
devil's bit 83
diaphrams 45
diet
    and choosing baby's sex 31
    fertility 50-4
    unborn baby 132-3
dietricians 52
Dong Quai 83
donor insemination 125
double spoons 26-7
Down's syndrome 13-14, 15
drink, alcohol 39, 47
drinking water 54
    filtering 54
drugs
    medication 71-4
    recreational 75
Duchenne muscular dystrophy 16
dwarfism 16

E

echinacea 85
ectopic pregnancies 21
eggs
    fertilization 20
    sperm penetration 19-20, 129
electrical appliances 69-70
electromagnetic fields, (EMFs) 64-5,
    69-70
embryo
    formation 21
    implantation 21-2
emotional health 42-3
endometriosis 115-16
enterococcus 49
ergotamine 72
Escherichia coli 49
essential fatty acids (EFAS) 51
essential oils 94-6
esters 94
eucalyptus, aromatherapy 94

exercise
men 46
women 37, 38

F
Fallopian tubes 19, 21
blocked 114–15
clearing blocked 127
stress and 59
false unicorn root 83
fat, body 37
feet, reflexology 97–9
Feng Shui 108–11
fennel, aromatherapy 95–6
ferning 118
fertile mucus 24
fertility
age and 12–16
five steps to 34
myths about 26–7
signs of 23–5
fertility day 10–11
fertilization 19–20
fibroids 116–17
homeopathy 80–1
fillings, teeth 55–8
fitness 38, 46
floorings, VOCs 69
flow cytometry 29
folic acid 51, 133
follicle-stimulating hormone (FSH) 15,
60, 126
food
and choosing baby's sex 31
detoxing 53–4
fertility 50–4
unborn baby 132–3
food intolerances 37
Foresight 34
formaldehyde 63, 67–8
fragile X syndrome 16
full moon 27, 28
furnishings, VOCs 69

G
Gamete intra-fallopian transfer (GIFT)
125, 127
gardening, dangerous chemicals 70
gardnerella 40, 49
gender pre-selection 28, 29–31
genetic counselling 16
genetic disorders, miscarriages 119
genetic problems, men 122
genetic testing 16
genito-urinary (GU) infections 36, 40
gentian 88
German chamomile 85
German measles
men 49
women 36, 40

GIFT 125, 127
GIFT-ET 127
ginger 85
girls, ways of choosing 28, 29–31
gonadotrophin-releasing analogues 126
gonadotrophin-releasing hormone
(GnRH) 126
gonorrhoea 49
grains 54
green vegetables 54
group B streptococci 49

H
haemolytic streptococci 49
haemophilia 16, 29
Haemophilus influenzae 49
hands, reflexology 97–9
health, preconceptual 33–75
heat, sperm and 48, 49, 122
helonias root 83
herbal medicines 74
herbalism 82–5, 74
herbicides 53, 63
heroin 75
herpes 49
HIV 41
home, health in the 67–70
homeopathy 78–81
honeysuckle 86
hormonal implant contraception 45
hormone replacement therapy (HRT),
male 15
hormones
male 14–15, 121–2, 128–9
miscarriages 119
houses, health and 67–70
human chorionic gonadotrophin (HCG)
22, 126
human menopausal gonadotrophin
(hMG) 126
hygiene 27
Hypericum perforatum 74
hypnotherapy 100–3, 105, 107

I
ICSI 125, 129
identical twins 20
impatiens 88–9
implantation 21–2
in-vitro fertilization (IVF) 34, 125, 127
costs 123
success rates 124
infections, miscarriages 119
infusions, herbalism 82
injections, contraceptive 45
insemination techniques 125
intercourse
best time for 10–11
positions and baby's sex 28
positions and fertility 26–7

intra-cytoplasmic sperm injection (ICSI)
129
intrauterine device (IUD) 44
intrauterine system (IUS) 44–5
iron 52
IUI 125
IVF 34, 125, 127
costs 123
success rates 124

K
Klebsiella 49

L
larch 88
lavender oil 96
law of similars 78
lead 63
libido, stress and 61–2
liferoot 84
lifestyle 119
lindane 68
lovemaking
best time for 10–11
positions and baby's sex 28
positions and fertility 26–7
luteinizing hormone (LH) 15, 25, 39

M
manganese 51
Marfan's syndrome 16
Matricaria chamomilla 85
medical infertility treatments 112–29
medication 71–4
preconceptual care 36
meditation 104, 105, 107
men
alcohol 47
body weight 46–7
exercise 46
fertility problems 120–2
herbal remedies 84–5
infections 49
medical treatments 128–9
preconceptual care 46–9
smoking 47–8
stress 60, 62
temperature 48, 49
menopause, smoking and 39
menstrual cycle
ovulation 24
ovulation day 10
menstruation
after fertilization 22
erratic periods 80
heavy periods 80
not having periods 80
mercury 63, 79
teeth fillings 55–8

methadone 75
metronidazole 72
mid-life crisis 14
minimum dose, homeopathy 78
miscarriages
    avoiding 133–4
    older fathers and 16
    older women 13
    repeated 118–19
    stress and 61
    VDUs and 64–5
    work-related hazards 63–4
missionary position 26
mitochondria 18
moon, full 27, 28
morphine 75
morula 21
mother cells 9
mucus, fertile 24
mycoplasma 40–1, 49

N
natural family planning (NFP) 44
Nei-Yi 92
neroli oil 96
nicotine patches 48, 72
non-identical twins 20
non-specific urethritis (NSU) 49
normal babies, older mothers 13–14
nuchal fold check 14
nutrition
    and choosing baby's sex 31
    fertility 50–4
    unborn baby 132–3
    supplements 52

O
o-day 10
oestrogen 61
    smoking and 39
oils, aromatherapy 94–5
older men
    age problems 15
    andropause 14–15
    and birth defects 15–16
    miscarriages and 16
older women
    fertility 12–13
    miscarriages 13
    normal babies 13–14
olive 88–9
opiates 75
orange oil 96
organic foods 53, 54
orgasms 28
ovarian cysts, homeopathy 80
ovulation 17
    cervix and 23
    encouraging 125–6
    pain 24

prediction kits 25
problems 114
signs of 24–5
ovulation day 10
oxytocin 60–1

P
paints, toxins 68–9
paracetamol 72
Passiflora incarnata 85
passionflower 85
passive muscle relaxation 106
peak fertility 10–11
pentoxifylline 128
periods
    erratic 80
    heavy 80
    homeopathy 80
    not having 80
    painful 80
permethrin 68
pesticides 53, 63
phenols 94
pheromones 23
pillows, love making 26
pine 88–9
pituitary gland 60
placentas 2
polycystic ovaries, homeopathy 80
polycystic ovary syndrome (POS) 115
post-coital test (PCT) 19, 117–18, 121
poultice tubes, herbalism 82
preconceptual care
    men 46–9
    women 7, 33–75
pregnancy 132–5
    tests 22
pro-fertility nutrients 50–2
progesterone 22, 39, 61
progestogen-only pill 44
prolactin 60
prostastitis 49
prostrate gland 18

R
rear entry, love making 26
reflexology 97–9
relaxation
    herbalism 85
    training 61
relaxation and visualization (R&V) 104–7
retinoids 72
retrograde ejaculation 121, 129
root vegetables 54
rose, aromatherapy 95
rubella
    men 49
    women, 36 40

S
St John's wort 74
Samana 83
saw palmetto 84
scent 23
schizophrenia 16
screen tests 40
selenium 50–1
semen 18–19
    analysis 120–1
    improving quality of 128
Senecio aureus 84
Serenoa serrulata 84
sex, baby's 28, 29–31
sex drive, stress and 61–2
sex positions
    and baby's sex 28
    and fertility 26–7
sexual energy, traditional Chinese
    medicine and 92
shift work 66
single remedies, homeopathy 78
sleeping pills 36
smoking
    men 47–8
    women 38–9
solvents 63, 64
sperm
    and baby's sex 29
    blocked tubes 129
    description 17–18
    faulty 16
    fertilization 20
    heat and 48, 49, 122
    improving quality 128
    and lifestyle 46
    passage to the egg 18–20, 27
    pre-selection 128
    saving 11
    semen analysis 120–1
sperm counts 120, 121
    improving 49, 128
    stress and 62, 122
spermicides 45
spina bifida 15, 51
Staphylococcus 49
star of Bethlehem 86
stress 59–62
    herbalism 85
    homeopathy 81
    men 60, 62
    sperm count 62, 122
symptothermal chart 24–5
synthetic vitamin A drugs 72

T
tea 54
teeth, fillings 55–8
temperature
    body 11
    men 48, 49

on ovulation 24-5
  sperm and 48, 49, 122
tense-release 106
teratogens 71
testicles, overheated 48, 49, 122
testosterone 14-15, 61, 62
thalidomide 72
trichomoniasis 40
thrush 25, 27
tinctures, herbalism 82
TINS 61-2
Tong Kuei 83
toxic substances
  in the home 67-70
  at work 63-4
toxic vapours 67-9
toxoplasmosis 40, 49
Traditional Chinese herbalism (TCH) 90, 91
tranquillizers 36, 72, 73
Turnera aphrodisiaca 84
twins 20

U
underweight, preconceptual 37
ureaplasma 40-1, 49
urine test 36

V
vagina, lubrication 23, 24
vaginal mucus 23, 24
varicoceles 48-9
VDUs 64-5
vegetables 54
vervain 88-9
vibration 66
viropause 14-15
visualization 104-7
vitamins 51-2
  B group 51
  C 51-2
  E 51
  supplements 52
Vitex agnus-castus 83
volatile organic compounds (VOCs) 67

W
water
  drinking 54
  filtering 53
weight
  men 46-7
  preconceptual 36-7
white chestnut 88-9
wild oat 85

wild rose 86
windows, pollution and 68
winter cherry 84
Withania omnifera 84
wombs
  implantation 21
  unusually-shaped 119
woodworm treatment 68
work environment 63-6
Wuzi Dihuang 92

X
X-carrying sperm 29, 30
xenoestrogens 53

Y
Y-carrying sperm 29, 30
ylang ylang 96
yoga 104
yohimbe 84

Z
Zibai Dihuang 92
zinc 50

Acknowledgements

Picture acknowledgements

Corbis UK Ltd/Bruce Burkhardt 91 bottom
/Dean Conger 97
/Bryan Cox 74
/Phil Schermeister 90
Getty Telegraph 10, 15, 35, 52, 61, 68, 70, 85 bottom, 96, 101, 112, 118, 122 bottom, 126, 134
Octopus Publishing Group Limited/Colin Bowling 82, 91 top
/Fiona Figoff 94 bottom
/Coling Gotts 8-9
/Andrew Lawson 87 top
/David Loftus 85 top, 108
/Peter Myers 95, 109
/Peter Pugh-Cook 29
/Bill Reavell 37, 76-77, 89, 100
/Simon Smith 30 top right, 51
/Ian Wallace 30 bottom left, 92, 93 left, 93 right, 98, 99, 104
/Mark Winwood 102 top, 105, 132
/Polly Wreford 110
Getty Image Bank 11, 12, 62, 75, 102 bottom, 106 top, 106 bottom, 124, 130, 133, 135
Photodisc 2-3, 6, 23, 32, 39, 41, 45, 46, 48, 50, 72
Science Photo Library 114
/Scot Camazine 58
/CNRI 119
/Manfred Kage 117
/James King-Holmes 122 top
/C.C. Kuo, University of Washington, Seattle 40
/Cordelia Molloy 86, 88
/Prof. P. Motta, Dept. of Anatomy, University 'La Sapienca', Rome 17, 18, 21
/Prof. P. Motta & S. Makabe 115
/Alfred Pasieka 57
/Chris Priest 127
/Quest 120
/Science Pictures Ltd. 73
/Volker Steger 78
/Dr. Yorgos Nicas 19, 22, 125
/Hattie Young 79
Getty Stone 13, 27, 38, 47, 59, 63, 64, 66 top, 66 bottom, 69, 80 top, 80 bottom, 81, 94 top

Author's acknowledgements

Especial thanks for their invaluable help and specialist knowledge go to:

Belinda Barnes, Director of the pioneering preconceptual care organization Foresight; the Colleges of Naturopathic & Complementary Medicine in East Grinstead, Belfast, Manchester and Dublin; environmental safety at work organization the London Hazards Centre; the national women's and children's HIV/AIDS support and campaigning group Positively Women; natural planning teaching organization Fertility UK; specialist family planning/fertility awareness GP and author Dr Karen Trewinnard and finally to Quicksilver Associates, New York.

Staff credits
Executive Editor Jane McIntosh
Editor Sharon Ashman
Design Manager Tokiko Morishima
Designer Mark Stevens
Picture Research Christine Junemann
Production Controller Viv Cracknell

Illustrations originally produced by Philip Wilson with additional amendments by Line + Line